Febrile Neutropenia

Febrile Neutropenia

Jean A Klastersky
Consultant, Medical Oncology
Institut Jules Bordet
Centre des Tumeurs de l'Universite Libre de Bruxelles
Brussels
Belgium

🐎 **Springer** Healthcare

Published by Springer Healthcare Ltd, 236 Gray's Inn Road, London, WC1X 8HB, UK.

www.springerhealthcare.com

British Library Cataloguing-in-Publication Data.

A catalogue record for this book is available from the British Library.

ISBN 9781907673696

Project editor: Tess Salazar
Production: Patty Goldstein
Printed in Great Britain by Latimer Trend

Contents

Author biography   vii

Abbreviations   viii

1   Introduction   **1**

Historical perspectives: why empirical therapy?   1

Current microbiological epidemiology   2

Common clinical presentations   6

Present achievements   7

Future directions   7

References   10

2   Prevention of febrile neutropenia   **13**

Risk factors predicting febrile neutropenia   13

Chemoprophylaxis   14

The use of granulopoietic colony stimulating   16

References   25

3   Prediction of the risk of complications associated with febrile neutropenia   **27**

Types and incidence of complications   27

Prediction of the individual risk of complications   28

Laboratory data and the Multinational Association of Supportive Cancer Care score index   29

The predictive value of the Multinational Association of Supportive Cancer Care index   31

References   34

4   Management of the low-risk patients   **35**

Orally administered antimicrobial therapy   35

Early hospital discharge   37

References   41

5 Management of the non-low-risk patients with febrile neutropenia   **43**

Predicting the non-low-risk patients with febrile neutropenia   43

Use of biological or microbiological parameters to predict poor outcome   44

Antibiotic management of non-low-risk patients   45

Non-low-risk patients at particular risk of septic complications   46

Follow-up and assessment of response   49

References   52

6 Management of persistent fever in patients with neutropenia despite empirical antibiotic administration   **55**

The causes of persistent fever   55

Prevention of invasive-fungal infection   56

Management of suspected invasive-fungal infection   57

Therapy of established invasive-fungal infections   60

References   61

7 Costs associated with febrile neutropenia   **63**

General conditions   63

Magnitude of the costs associated with febrile neutropenia   63

Reducing the cost of febrile neutropenia   64

References   68

8 At the extremes of age: febrile neutropenia in children and elderly   **69**

Febrile neutropenia in the pediatric population   69

Febrile neutropenia in the elderly   70

References   73

Author biography

Jean A Klastersky, MD, PhD, is head of the Department of Medicine at the Institut Jules Bordet in Brussels and has been Professor of Medicine, Medical Oncology, and Physical Diagnosis at the Université Libre de Bruxelles since 1977.

Professor Klastersky was an Intern and Resident at the University Hospitals of the Université Libre de Bruxelles between 1962 and 1965 where he gained his MD (Docteur en Médecine, Chirurgie et Accouchements). From 1967 to 1968 he was Chief-Resident at Boston City Hospital and then a Research Fellow and Assistant in Medicine at Thorndike Memorial Laboratory, Harvard Medical School. He became Chief of the Section of Infectious Diseases at the Institut Jules Bordet in 1970 before taking up his current position in 1977.

Professor Klastersky was a founder member of the European Lung Cancer Working Party and has been its President since 1978. He was President (and founding member) of the International European Organisation for Research and Treatment of Cancer (EORTC) Antimicrobial Therapy Project Group between 1979 and 1987 and the Group's Secretary General from 1987 to 2000. He was President (and founding member) of the Multinational Association for Supportive Care in Cancer (MASCC) from 1990 to 2000, and has been Visiting Professor of Medical Oncology at Charles University, Prague since 1994.

Professor Klastersky is a member of the American Society of Clinical Oncology, the American Association of Cancer Research, the European Society of Medical Oncology, the American Society of Microbiology, the Infectious Disease Society of America, the International Association for the Study of Lung Cancer, and various other international and national medical and/or oncological societies.

Abbreviations

ANC	absolute neutrophil count
ASCO	American Society of Clinical Oncology
BCG	Bacillus Calmette–Guérin
CNS	central nervous system
CRP	C-reactive protein
CT	computed tomography
ECOG	Eastern Cooperative Oncology Group
EORTC	European Organisation for Research and Treatment of Cancer
ESMO	European Society of Medical Oncology
FAC	fluorouracil, doxorubicin, cyclophosphamide
FN	febrile neutropenia
FUO	fever of unknown origin
G-CSF	granulocyte colony-stimulating factor
ID	infectious disease
IDSA	Infectious Diseases Society of America
IFD	invasive-fungal diseases
IL	interleukin
MASCC	Multinational Association for Supportive Care in Cancer
PCR	polymerase chain reaction
Pros	prospective study
RCT	randomized clinical trial
Retro	retrospective study
SMX	sulfamethoxazole
TAC	docetaxel, doxorubicin, cyclophosphamide
TMP	trimethoprim
VZV	varicella-zoster virus

Chapter 1

Introduction

Historical perspectives: why empirical therapy?

The relationship between neutropenia and the risk of severe infection in patients with cancer has been clearly established early in the 1960s by Bodey et al [1]. At that time, Gram-negative bacteremia in neutropenic patients with cancer (most often with acute leukemia) carried an exceedingly high mortality of 90% [2]. More specifically, it was shown that sepsis due to *Pseudomonas aeruginosa* or *Escherichia coli* was lethal in about half of cases within 48 hours after the first blood culture had been taken [3]. Moreover, it was demonstrated that infection in patients with neutropenia was associated with few obvious signs and symptoms of infection and was often associated with bacteremia [4]. The difficulty in documenting infection and/or bacteremia led to the idea of administering broad-spectrum antimicrobial therapy to patients with febrile neutropenia (FN) as soon as fever developed without waiting for further microbiological or clinical evidence of infection. Thus, two important concepts have emerged at that time: first, the "syndrome" of FN as a surrogate for potential severe infection in chemotherapy-treated patients with cancer and, second, a paradigm of therapy: empirical broad-spectrum antimicrobial therapy. The importance of these two concepts, developed more than 50 years ago, has never been challenged and is still valid today. Although the concept of empirical therapy for FN has never been validated in a prospective controlled clinical study, it gained

J. A. Klastersky, *Febrile Neutropenia*,
DOI: 10.1007/978-1-907673-70-2_1, © Springer Healthcare 2014

wide acceptance based on its obvious efficacy. On the other hand, the type of empirical therapy to be used has been the target of many studies.

Current microbiological epidemiology

In the early 1960s and 1970s, Gram-negative bacilli, namely *P. aeruginosa* and *E. coli*, were the most frequently associated pathogens with FN. This probably explains why potentially synergistic combinations against these pathogens proved to be particularly effective; early studies supported the concept of anti-Gram-negatives oriented empirical therapy [5,6] and suggested reasons for the use of synergistic combinations of antibiotics [7]. Today, evidence has been provided for the efficacy of monotherapy that seems to be as effective as combination therapy [8], making the need for synergistic combinations of antibiotics less important than hitherto. Whether this is a consequence of the development of more potent antibiotics and/or results from improvements in oncological and supportive care of patients with cancer remains unclear so far.

As shown in Table 1.1, Gram-positive microorganisms became more frequently isolated in cases of FN in the late 1980s and were the most common pathogens in the 1990s [9]. These microbiological changes have multiple causes, such as the frequent use of permanent intravenous devices (predisposing patients to infections by the coagulase-negative staphylococci) and the prescription of prophylactic antimicrobials to prevent FN, namely sulfamethoxazole-trimethoprim and later the fluoroquinolones (predisposing patients to infections by streptococcal species). There has been a significant reduction of the incidence of Gram-negative infections with the use of such a prophylaxis, at the cost of the emergence of resistance not only to the agents used for prophylaxis but also to other classes of antimicrobials, as will be discussed later [10]. The Gram-positive infections, namely those caused by coagulase-negative staphylococci, are associated with much lower rates of morbidity and mortality than infections caused by Gram-negative rods. Therefore, the addition of glycopeptides to empirical regimens aimed to cover Gram negatives is probably not necessary; the streptococci are usually covered by the antibiotics used for anti-Gram-negative coverage [11,12].

Bacteremia in clinical trials of the European Organisation for Research and Treatment of Cancer International Antimicrobial Therapy Cooperative Group

Trial	Period	No. of patients	Single-organism bacteremia	
			% Gram-negative	% Gram-positive
I	1973–1976	145	71	29
II	1977–1980	111	67	23
III	1980–1983	141	59	41
IV	1983–1985	219	59	41
V	1986–1988	213	37	63
VIII	1989–1991	151	31	69
IX	1991–1993	161	33	67
XI	1994–1996	199	31	69
XII (low risk)	1995–1997	39	59	41
XIV (high risk)	1997–2000	186	47	53

Table 1.1 Bacteremia in clinical trials of the European Organisation for Research and Treatment of Cancer International Antimicrobial Therapy Cooperative Group. Reproduced with permission from © Taylor and Francis 2013, Kern [9]. All Rights Reserved.

The respective distribution of Gram-positive and Gram-negative pathogens in patients with FN today is illustrated in Table 1.2, summarizing a large retrospective review of patients with FN [13]. It can be seen that Gram positives represented 57% of the infections and Gram negatives were responsible for 34%. The rates of serious complications or death were respectively 20% and 5% for Gram-positive infections and 23% and 18% for Gram-negative infections, confirming earlier epidemiological and prognostic features that have a role in defining optimal therapy.

Whether bacterial infection is responsible for most initial episodes of FN, persisting fever in patients with neutropenia, not responding to initial empirical therapy, is often associated with fungal infection, especially in patients with protracted neutropenia; the incidence of fungal infections, under these circumstances, might be as high as 30% [14]. Empirical therapy with various antifungal regimens (liposomal amphotericin B, voriconazole, or caspofungin) has been associated with favorable results, especially since the early diagnosis of fungal infection can be difficult and the mortality associated with disseminated fungal infection in patients with neutropenia is very high [15].

Incidence of causative pathogens and outcome according to microbiology

	Total	Incidence
Single GM−	**168**	
Acinetobacter	4	2%
Aeromonas hydrophila	1	<1%
Bacteroides	3	2%
Capnocytophaga	3	2%
Citrobacter	1	<1%
Enterobacter	7	4%
Escherichia coli	72	41%
Fusobacterium	7	4%
GM− rod	1	<1%
Haemophilus	1	<1%
Klebsiella	20	11%
Morganella	1	<1%
Proteus	2	1%
Pseudomonas	42	24%
Serratia	1	<1%
Stenotrophomonas	1	<1%
Xanothomonas	1	<1%
Single GM+	**283**	
Bacillus	6	2%
Clostridium	4	1%
Corynebacterium	8	3%
Coryneform bacteria	4	1%
Enterococcus	8	5%
Lactobacillus	1	<1%
Micrococcus species	1	<1%
Peptostreptocossus	1	<1%
Pneumococcus	1	<1%
Propionibacterium	3	1%
Staphylococcus (coag −)	138	50%
Staphylococcus (coag +)	25	9%
Stomatococcus	10	4%
Streptococcus	73	27%
Polymicrobial	**48**	
Containing at least one GM− organism	29	60%
Containing only GM+ organisms	19	40%

Table 1.2 Incidence of causative pathogens and outcome according to microbiology (continues over). GM−, Gram-negative; GM+, Gram-positive. The complications rate and death rate were only calculated in subgroups of more than 10 cases.

	Complications (non-lethal)		Death	
Single GM−	**38**	**23%**	**30**	**18%**
Acinetobacter	1		−	
Aeromonas hydrophila	1		−	
Bacteroides	−		1	
Capnocytophaga	−		1	
Citrobacter	−		−	
Enterobacter	−		−	
Escherichia coli	19	26%	13	18%
Fusobacterium	−		−	
GM− rod	−		−	
Haemophilus	1		−	
Klebsiella	6	30%	2	10%
Morganella	−		−	
Proteus	−		−	
Pseudomonas	8	19%	13	31%
Serratia	1		−	
Stenotrophomonas	1		−	
Xanothomonas	−		−	
Single GM+	**57**	**20%**	**13**	**5%**
Bacillus	1		1	
Clostridium	1		−	
Corynebacterium	3		−	
Coryneform bacteria	1		−	
Enterococcus	2		−	
Lactobacillus	1		−	
Micrococcus species	−		−	
Peptostreptocossus	−		−	
Pneumococcus	−		1	
Propionibacterium	−		−	
Staphylococcus (coag −)	21	15%	8	6%
Staphylococcus (coag +)	6	24%	−	−
Stomatococcus	2		−	
Streptococcus	19	26%	3	4%
Polymicrobial	**11**	**23%**	**6**	**13%**
Containing at least one GM− organism	8	28%	5	17%
Containing only GM+ organisms	3	16%	1	5%

Table 1.2 Incidence of causative pathogens and outcome according to microbiology (continued). Reproduced with permission from © Elsevier 2013, Klastersky et al [13]. All Rights Reserved.

Common clinical presentations

Bacteremia is a frequent clinical presentation of infection in patients with FN; it occurs in about 20–30% of patients with FN and carries a rate of complications and death higher than that in nonbacteremic patients with FN. As already mentioned, Gram-positive and Gram-negative microorganisms are currently responsible for about 50% of the bacteremic episodes each with different consequences in terms of morbidity and mortality.

The question of the microbiological nature of the nonbacteremic episodes of FN is difficult to answer; yet, the vast majority of patients respond with prompt defervescence and clinical improvement to empirical antimicrobial therapy, suggesting that occult bacterial infection is present in most of the cases [16].

Clinically localized infections in patients with FN are probably underestimated since severe neutropenia may minimize clinical signs and symptoms of infection, namely inflammatory changes. The demonstration of a potential clinical site of an infection during FN does not modify the overall therapeutic strategy. Nonetheless, the demonstration of a localized infection should be an incentive to obtain specific material for microbiological investigations, in addition to blood cultures, in order to better and earlier define a possible pathogen, as this may lead to an adaptation of the initial antimicrobial therapy. Moreover, the presence of a localized infection often poses the question of surgical drainage and/or removal of a foreign body (eg, catheter), if feasible.

The presence of clinically apparent sites of infection (eg, pneumonia, urinary tract infection, neutropenic enterocolitis, perirectal infection), which are usually polymicrobial or predominantly Gram negative, is often considered to have a higher morbidity/mortality than simple bacteremia [17]. It is possible that these "complicated" bacteremias correspond to a later stage of infection than FN associated with "simple" bacteremia. Since the microbiological cause of the fever in nonbacteremic cases may be less obvious than in bacteremic cases, it is difficult to compare the prognosis and the outcome of these patients to those with documented bacteremia, with or without the presence of a clinical site of possible infection. Nevertheless, pneumonia represents one of the most critical infections in patients with FN whether it is associated with bacteremia or not. Patients who develop respiratory insufficiency have a poor prognosis; only 20% or less survive.

Although chest computed tomography (CT) scans have substantially improved the diagnostic sensitivity and specificity for pulmonary infections during FN, the precise etiology can be defined in less than 50% of cases partly because patients have often been given empirical therapy and because invasive diagnostic procedures (bronchoscopy, broncho–alveolar lavage, lung biopsy) are often difficult to perform due to the frail condition of the patients and/or thrombocytopenia. Therefore, special attention should be paid to selective clinical signs or symptoms that could orient the clinician towards a specific diagnosis as well as to serological and other nonmicrobiological clues (Table 1.3) [18].

Present achievements

This book will focus on the present day paradigms for the management of FN. A series of standard attitudes have been developed and will be discussed here, although it should be clear that these recommendations are in a constant state of evolution and need to be adapted to the progresses in cancer management and improvements in supportive care.

The major issues that will be dealt with here have been recently reviewed [19] and are summarized in Table 1.4.

Future directions

Where do we go from here? As indicated in Table 1.5 [19], the changing nature and sensitivity of the offending pathogens may require the development of broader and more potent antibiotics, although there is little evidence that this will happen in a near future. As some of the complications and death in patients with FN do occur in spite of the use of adequate antimicrobial therapy, it might be essential to pay more attention to the pathology of severe sepsis during FN. Another approach might be the development of cancer therapies that would be less inductive of neutropenia and immunosuppression.

Finally, as the use of empirical strategies reflects our limited ability to rapidly and precisely diagnose the microbiological causes of infections during FN, progress in microbiological diagnosis might lead to a more

Pathogens causing pulmonary infections, with predisposing factors, clinical patterns, and recommended therapy (continues over)

Pathogen	Predisposing factors	Sources	Recommended therapy
P. carinii	Cellular immunity	Subacute onset, dyspnea, hypoxia, interstitial pulmonary infiltrates	TMP-SMX pentamidine or TMP-dapsone
Aspergillus spp.	Neutropenia	Acute onset, pleuritic chest pain, cutaneous ulcerations (rare), CNS abscesses, solitary or multiple nodular lesions on X-ray with halo sign or cavitation	Amphotericin B
Mucorales	Neutropenia	Acute onset and fulminant course, palatal necrotic ulcer, radiography findings similar to aspergillosis	Amphotericin B
Coccidioides spp.	Cellular immunity	Travel to endemic area, acute progressive peumonia with miliary dissemination	Amphotericin B
Histoplasma capsulatum	Cellular immunity	Hepatosplenomegaly, patchy infiltrates, miliary dissemination, chest radiograph may be normal	Amphotericin B, ketoconazole, or itraconazole can be given for moderate disease
Fusarium and *P. boydii*	Neutropenia	Similar to aspergillosis with more frequent cutaneous ulceration, both can be isolated from blood	Both invariably resistant to amphotericin B, no standard therapy for *Fusarium*, miconazole for *P. boydii*
Mycobacterium tuberculosis	Cellular immunity	History of previous disease or contact, chronic course, cavitations in upper lobes, rarely miliary	Isoniazid and rifampicin for 6 months, pyrazinamide for 2 months
Legionella spp.	Cellular immunity	Acute onset, hypoxia, extrapulmonary manifestations such as diarrhea and confusion, unilobar or multilobar consolidation	Combined erythromycin and rifampicin, or a fluoroquinolone plus rifampicin
Nocardia spp.	Cellular immunity	Chronic onset, nodular subcutaneous lesions, brain abscesses, solitary or multiple cavitations, reticulonodular infiltrates and empyema, upper lobes commonly involved	TMP-SMX or a sulphonamide
Rhodococcus equi	Cellular immunity	Animal contacts, cavitations in upper lobes	Combined erythromycin and rifampicin

Table 1.3 Pathogens causing pulmonary infections, with predisposing factors, clinical patterns, and recommended therapy (continues over).

Pathogens causing pulmonary infections, with predisposing factors, clinical patterns, and recommended therapy (continued)

Pathogen	Predisposing factors	Sources	Recommended therapy
Strongyloides stercoralis	Cellular immunity	Urticaria and pruritus, gastrointestinal symptoms, diffuse alveolar infiltrates, eosinophilia may be absent in 50% of immunosuppressed patients	Thiabendazole
Cytomegalovirus	Cellular immunity	Subacute onset, hypoxia, interstitial pneumonia, often in recipients of bone marrow transplants	Ganciclovir
Herpes simplex and herpes zoster-varicella viruses	Cellular immunity	Subacute onset, mucosal, and cutaneous lesions may precede pneumonia (interstitial, focal, or multifocal)	Acyclovir
Adenovirus	Cellular immunity	Subacute conjunctivitis, hematuria, diffuse interstitial pneumonia, pleural effusion	No therapy
Respiratory syncytial virus	Cellular immunity	Subacute onset, upper respiratory symptoms, bilateral diffuse infiltrates	Ribavirin?

Table 1.3 Pathogens causing pulmonary infections, with predisposing factors, clinical patterns, and recommended therapy. CNS, central nervous system; SMX, sulfamethoxazole; TMP, trimethoprim. Reproduced with permission from © Oxford University Press 2013, Klastersky, Aoun [18]. All Rights Reserved.

Standard approaches for the management of febrile neutropenia

1.	Prevention (antibiotics and/or CSFs) is essential
2.	Empirical therapy remains a basic rule
3.	Antimicrobial therapy and overall management can be adjusted to the risk of complications
4.	Antimicrobial monotherapy is adequate in most cases but early and rational changes are often needed
5.	Occult fungal infection must be suspected in patients with protracted febrile neutropenia and be managed with empirical pre-emptive antifungal therapy

Table 1.4 Standard approaches for the management of febrile neutropenia. CSF, colony-stimulating factor. Reproduced with permission from © Elsevier 2013, Klastersky et al [19]. All Rights Reserved.

Future possible avenues to cope with febrile neutropenia	
1.	Development of more potent antibiotics
2.	Intensive care of severe sepsis
3.	Less aggressive anticancer regimens
4.	More specific and earlier laboratory microbiological diagnosis
5.	Use of biomarkers for infection
6.	Imaging techniques

Table 1.5 Future possible avenues to cope with febrile neutropenia. Reproduced with permission from © Elsevier 2013, Klastersky et al [19]. All Rights Reserved.

selective and specific use of antimicrobials. Newer laboratory markers might also improve our capability of coping with FN, especially in high-risk patients. In addition, imaging techniques with high resolution CT scanners at magnetic resonance imaging may help with early and more specific diagnosis as well as with better evaluation of response to therapy [20].

References

1 Bodey GP. The changing face of febrile neutropenia-from monotherapy to moulds to mucositis. Fever and neutropenia: the early years. *J Antimicrob Chemother.* 2009;63:i3-13.

2 McCabe W, Jackson G. Gram-negative bacteremia: II. clinical, laboratory and therapeutic observations. *Arch Intern Med.* 1962;110:856-864.

3 Bodey GP, Jadeja L, Elting L. Retrospective analysis of 410 episodes of Pseudomonas bacteremia. *Arch Intern Med.* 1985;145:1621-1629.

4 Sickles EA, Green WH, et al. Clinical presentation in granulopoietic patients. *Arch Intern Med.* 1975;135:715-719.

5 Schimpff S, Satterlee W, Young VM, Serpick A. Empiric therapy with carbenicillin and gentamicin for febrile patients with cancer and granulocytopenia. *N Engl J Med.* 1971;284:1061-1065.

6 Klastersky J, Cappel R, Debusscher L. Evaluation of gentamicin with carbenicillin in infections due to gram-negative bacilli. *Curr Ther Res Clin Exp.* 1971;13:174-781.

7 Klastersky J. Empiric treatment of infections in neutropenic patients with cancer. *Rev Infect Dis.* 1983;5:S21-S31.

8 Paul M, Soares-Weiser K, Leibovici L. Beta lactam monotherapy versus beta-lactam aminoglycoside combination therapy for fever with neutropenia: systematic review and meta-analysis. *BMJ.* 2003;326:1111.

9 Kern WV. Current epidemiology in of infections in neutropenic cancer patients. In: Rolston RV, Rubinstein EB, eds *Textbook of Febrile Neutropenia.* London, UK: Martin Dunitz, Ltd; 2001:57-90.

10 Cattaneo C, Quaresmini G, Casari S, et al. Recent changes in bacterial epidemiology and the emergence of fluoroquinolone-resistant Escherichia coli among patients with haematological malignancies: results of a prospective study on 823 patients at a single institution. *J Antimicrob Chemother.* 2008;61:721-728.

11 Vancomycin added to empirical combination antibiotic therapy for fever in granulocytopenic cancer patients. European Organization for Research and Treatment of Cancer (EORTC) International Antimicrobial Therapy Cooperative Group and the National Cancer Institute of Canada-Clinical Trials Group. *J Infect Dis.* 1991;163:951-958.

12 Cometta A, Kern WV, De Bock R, et al; International Antimicrobial Therapy Group of the European Organization for Research Treatment of Cancer. Vancomycin versus placebo for treating persistent fever in patients with neutropenic cancer receiving piperacillin-tazobactam monotherapy. *Clin Infect Dis.* 2003;37:382-389.

13 Klastersky J, Ameye L, Maertens J, et al. Bacteremia in febrile neutropenic cancer patients. *Int J Antimicrob Agents.* 2007;30:S51-S59.

14 Corey L, Boeckh M. Persistent fever in patients with neutropenia. *N Engl J Med.* 2002;346:222-224.

15 Klastersky J. Antifungal therapy in patients with fever and neutropenia--more rational and less empirical? *N Engl J Med.* 2004;351:1445-1447.

16 Schimpff SC, Gaya H, Klastersky J, Tattersall MH, Zinner SH. Three antibiotic regimens in the treatment of infection in febrile granulocytopenic patients with cancer. The EORTC international antimicrobial therapy project group. *J Infect Dis.* 1978;137:14-29.

17 Elting LS, Rubenstein EB, Rolston KV, Bodey GP. Outcomes of bacteremia in patients with cancer and neutropenia: observations from two decades of epidemiological and clinical trials. *Clin Infect Dis.* 1997;25:247-259.

18 Klastersky J, Aoun M. Opportunistic infections in patients with cancer. *Ann Oncol.* 2004;15(Suppl 4):iv329-iv335.

19 Klastersky J, Awada A, Paesmans M, Aoun M. Febrile Neutropenia: A critical review of the initial management. *Crit Rev Oncol Hematol.* 2011;78:185-194.

20 Rieger C, Herzog P, Eibel R, Fiegl M, Ostermann H. Pulmonary MRI – a new approach for the evaluation of febrile neutropenic patients with malignancies. *Support Care Cancer.* 2008;16:599-606.

Chapter 2

Prevention of febrile neutropenia

Risk factors predicting febrile neutropenia

As infection in patients with neutropenia is primarily the direct consequence of chemotherapy-induced neutropenia, attempts to prevent febrile
neutropenia (FN) episodes during chemotherapy administration requires
the evaluation of the risk factors associated with the development of
significant neutropenia.

Neutropenia in chemotherapy-treated patients with solid tumors is
related to the intensity of the administered chemotherapy and, consequently, most common chemotherapy regimens have been associated with
a predictable risk of FN [1]. However, this prediction is far from being
highly accurate, as other patient-related risk factors should be taken into
account, in addition to the intensity of chemotherapy. Particular consideration should be given to the elevated risk of FN in elderly patients
(aged 65 and over). Other adverse risk factors that may influence FN risk
include: advanced stage of disease, experience of previous episodes of
FN, lack of prophylaxis (granulocyte colony-stimulating factor [G-CSF]
use or antibiotic prophylaxis) as well as the use of concomitant immu-
nosuppressive agents or various serious comorbidities, such as diabetes,
cirrhosis, and others.

In patients with hematological malignancies, it has been confirmed
that an aggressive chemotherapy regimen was the major predictor of
FN. Other independent predictors were the underlying disease, the
involvement of the bone marrow, a body surface ≤2 m^2, and a baseline

J. A. Klastersky, *Febrile Neutropenia*,
DOI: 10.1007/978-1-907673-70-2_2, © Springer Healthcare 2014

monocyte count <150/µl [2]. Many other attempts have been made to predict the occurrence of FN and several predictive factors have been proposed, such as the slope of the myelosuppression-time profile [3] or the type of cancer and renal function tests [4], but further prospective validation is needed.

Based on these different risk factors, models have been proposed to better predict the occurrence of FN in patients treated with chemotherapy, and consequently provide the greatest clinical benefit and cost effective use of prophylaxis [5]. However, so far none of these models have gained wide acceptance and/or have been validated in large prospective trials.

While elderly patients clearly have a higher rate of complications during FN than younger patients treated with similar regimens [6], in children the aggressiveness of chemotherapy and the level of neutropenia at the onset of FN appear to be the strongest risk factors associated with the development of FN [7].

Chemoprophylaxis

Attempts had been made 50 years ago to reduce the occurrence of FN in high-risks patients (ie, those with acute leukemia aggressively treated with chemotherapy) with the implementation of a protective environment (eg, isolation and the use of low-bacterial diet) in combination with orally administered nonabsorbable antibiotics. Overall, these approaches have been disappointing in terms of efficacy and tolerability by the patients. Moreover, recent reviews stressed the essential role of orally administered antibiotics compared to the other components of the protective environment, namely isolation and low-bacterial diet [8]; on the other hand, oral-nonabsorbable antibiotics given to leukemia patients within protective environments have been associated with the emergence of resistant strains [9]. For all these reasons, the protective environment approach has been largely abandoned.

The prophylactic oral administration of absorbable antibiotics has been initially successful with the use of co-trimoxazole. However, the emergence of co-trimoxazole-resistant strains rapidly limited the clinical effectiveness of that approach [10].

More recently, fluoroquinolones have been used for the prevention of FN in patients treated with chemotherapy, with either solid or hematological malignancies. Meta-analyses indicated that such an antimicrobial prophylaxis reduced the frequency of infection and infection-related mortality in neutropenic patients with cancer [11] but led to the emergence of quinolone-resistant strains that could be resistant to a wide spectrum of antibiotics [12]. It should be emphasized that the favorable results of the prophylactic fluoroquinolones has been mainly observed in patients with a high risk of FN (ie, patients treated for acute leukemia and/or receiving hematopoietic stem cell transplantation); for the patients with a low risk for FN, the evidence that antibacterial prophylaxis improves the outcome is less robust. Based on these considerations and because the routine use of antibacterial prophylaxis may increase the spread of resistant strains, recent guidelines from the American Society of Clinical Oncology (ASCO) recommend that clinicians limit the use of antibacterial prophylaxis to patients at high risk for FN [13]. Nonetheless, others recommend the mere avoidance of prophylactic use of fluoroquinolones for the prevention of FN. First, the use of fluoroquinolones for prophylaxis will eventually make that approach useless, as a result of the emergence of resistant strains, just as it has been the case with trimethoprim-sulfamethoxazole. Next, the emergence of fluoroquinolone resistance might be associated with a worse outcome of bacteremia, through the emergence of multiresistance, and that situation would require new paradigms in terms of empirical therapy. Finally, fluoroquinolone prophylaxis makes the empirical therapy of FN based on fluoroquinolones impossible [14], although in patients not previously exposed to quinolones such an approach has been shown to be highly effective [15]. For all these reasons, it would appear sensible to discontinue the prophylactic use of fluoroquinolones in patients with cancer.

These recommendations are supported by recent evidence obtained in the pediatric population (in which the quinolones are usually not used because of their possible interference with bone metabolism). Although ciprofloxacin significantly reduced the occurrence of FN in children with acute lymphoblastic leukemia in the induction phase of chemotherapy, the percentage of *Escherichia coli* and *Klebsiella pneumoniae* susceptible to ciprofloxacin were significantly lower in the patients having received ciprofloxacin [16].

Besides antibacterial prophylaxis, as indicated in Table 2.1, antiviral and antifungal prophylactic measures need to be considered for patients with prolonged neutropenia and/or severe immunodepression, namely in patients undergoing hematopoietic stem cell transplantation [17]. In those patients, vaccination programs should avoid live vaccines as long as the immunologic recovery as not complete.

The use of granulopoietic colony stimulating

The development of the G-CSFs provided oncologists a much more physiological way to prevent chemotherapy-associated FN, compared with chemoprophylaxis.

Primary prophylaxis

In 2007, Kuderer et al published a comprehensive systematic review and meta-analysis of all reported randomized controlled trials comparing

Antibacterial prophylaxis		
Modality	**Patient group**	**Treatment**
Vaccination		Yearly influenza vaccine 5-year pneumococcal vaccine No live vaccines (eg, oral polio, oral typhoid, yellow fever, measles, mumps, rubella, BCG, VZV
Antibacterial	Patients undergoing intensive chemotherapy and expected to present a prolonged and profound neutropenia (ANC <100 cells/mm³ for more than 7 days)	Ciprofloxacin Levofloxacin
Antiviral	Patients with recurrent herpes infections undergoing intensive chemotherapy and expected to present a prolonged and profound neutropenia; lymphopenic patients	Acyclovir Valacyclovir
Antifungal	Patients undergoing intensive chemotherapy and expected to present a prolonged and profound neutropenia	Fluconazole Posaconazole Itraconazole

Table 2.1 Antibacterial prophylaxis. ANC, absolute neutrophil count; BCG, Bacillus Calmette–Guérin; VZV, varicella-zoster virus. Reproduced with permission from © Marcel Decker 2013, Bron [17]. All Rights Reserved.

G-CSF with placebo or untreated controls in adults with solid tumors or lymphomas [18]. The most important conclusions were a significant reduction of the infection-related mortality (from 2.8% to 1.5%) and a significant reduction of FN episodes (from 39% to 22%), impacting morbidity and cost of care. Moreover, the relative dose intensity was clearly higher in the patients receiving G-CSF: 90–99% in patients receiving G-CSF versus 71–95% in the control groups, suggesting that dose reductions and delays in the administration of chemotherapy had been reduced.

More recently, another systematic review and meta-analysis reported similar results [19]. Overall, it was found that the relative risk of FN for G-CSF prophylaxis versus no primary prophylaxis was 0.51 in patients with solid tumors and lymphomas.

In patients treated with high-dose chemotherapy followed by stem cell transplantation, another recent meta-analysis showed that G-CSF reduced the risk of documented infections and time to hematologic recovery as well as the duration of hospital stay [20]. However, there was no difference between G-CSF treatment group and placebo group for all-cause mortality.

Based on these data G-CSF primary prophylaxis significantly reduces the morbidity resulting from FN, improves the quality of life of the patients, possibly makes chemotherapy more efficacious, and the overall management of the patients less expensive. The effect on FN and mortality has been extensively discussed in the literature, as indicated in Figure 2.1 [21].

Secondary prophylaxis

Secondary prophylaxis is the administration of G-CSF to patients who already experienced an episode of FN during a previous cycle of chemotherapy; it has been less studied than primary prophylaxis.

The initial G-CSF registration study in patients with small cell lung cancer receiving intensive chemotherapy allowed patients in the placebo group to receive open-label G-CSF in subsequent cycles of chemotherapy after an FN episode during the first cycle. The secondary prophylaxis in those patients, all of whom had experienced FN during the first cycle,

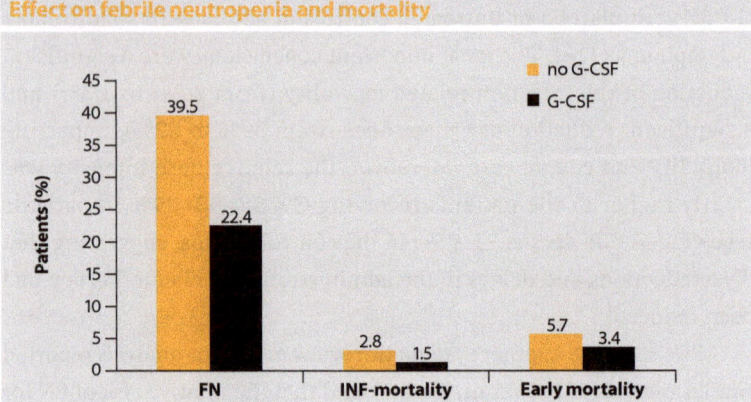

Figure 2.1 Effect on febrile neutropenia and mortality. Efficacy of primary prophylactic G-CSF (pegfilgrastim, filgrastim, or lenograstim) versus placebo or no treatment in preventing febrile neutropenia, INF-related mortality, and early mortality (all-cause, during chemotherapy) in 3493 patients treated with chemotherapy for solid tumors or lymphoma. Results of a meta-analysis of 17 studies. FN, febrile neutropenia; G-CSF, granulocyte colony-stimulating factor; INF, infection. Reproduced with permission from © Springer-Verlag 2013, Aapro et al [21]. All Rights Reserved.

was associated with FN in only 23% [22]. Similar results were presented in a more recent investigation in 48 patients with different tumors and therapies and who all developed an FN episode during the first cycle of chemotherapy. These patients received G-CSF during the subsequent course of the same chemotherapy without any reduction of the dose intensity; with secondary prophylaxis the frequency of FN was 2% (one patient out of 48) [23]. The level of the reduction of the risk of FN with secondary prophylaxis is probably influenced by factors, such as the type of tumor and chemotherapy; it might be greater with less aggressive regimens. Those two studies showed a dramatic reduction of FN with secondary prophylaxis; however, it should be recognized that the risk of FN has been found greatest during the initial treatment cycle [24].

Another study [25] reported the results of a randomized trial comparing adjuvant docetaxel, doxorubicin, cyclophosphamide (TAC) and fluorouracil, doxorubicin, cyclophosphamide (FAC) for high-risk cancer patients; the study indicated that secondary prophylaxis was effective but also suggested that with regimens associated with a high risk of

FN (TAC), primary prophylaxis should be the rule as the frequency of FN was still 24% with secondary prophylaxis while only 6% with the primary approach.

The choice of granulocyte colony-stimulating factor for primary prophylaxis

At the present time, there are two preparations of G-CSF available for clinical use. Filgrastim is eliminated by the renal route as well as inactivation by the rising number of neutrophils, and requires a daily administration until neutrophil recovery. The other is a long-acting preparation, obtained by pegylation: pegfilgrastim is inactivated by the stimulated neutrophils a few days after its administration, and thus only needs a single administration.

There have been numerous studies comparing these two preparations and the optimal ways for their administration [26]. Recent reviews suggest that pegfilgrastim might be associated with a lower risk of FN-related hospitalization of patients with solid tumors than filgrastim prophylaxis [27]. In patients treated with intensive chemotherapy and autologous peripheral stem cell transplantation, recent reports state that both drugs are at least equally effective [28]. There are no indications that one of these preparations is safer than the other; both can be associated with some bone pain but serious complications are extremely rare.

The choice between the use of pegfilgrastim or filgrastim may take into account the convenience of administration of pegfilgrastim (a single injection) and the lower cost of filgrastim, especially if reduced schedules of administration and the use of less expensive biosimilars are taken into consideration.

Guidelines for selecting patients for granulocyte colony-stimulating factor prophylaxis

All of the published guidelines about the use of G-CSF for the prophylaxis of FN estimate risk for developing FN based on the type of chemotherapy used. Although there are lists of chemotherapy regimens with an estimation of the risk of FN associated, respectively [1], there is no validated tool for categorizing chemotherapy regimens according to their toxicity on the neutrophils. Moreover, various comorbidities might significantly increase the risk of FN, for a given regimen, namely age.

All published guidelines use a three-step classification with three categories: high risk of developing FN (ie, >20%), intermediate risk (10–20%), and low risk (<10%). The underlying drive is cost effectiveness, a delicate balance between the savings resulting from effective prevention of FN and the cost of G-CSF.

All guidelines recommend using G-CSF if the risk of FN is greater than 20% (the high-risk group) but diverge as far as the other groups are concerned; however, there might be a consensus for not giving prophylaxis with G-CSF to patients with a lower than 10% risk of developing FN.

The recommendations made by European Organisation for Research and Treatment of Cancer (EORTC) in 2010 [1] represent a pragmatic approach and are summarized in Figure 2.2 [1]. Although these guidelines adopt the three-step approach, common to all published recommendations so far, they provide a significant space for the role of various comorbidities in the decision planning. This is a very important step towards a more precisely tailored approach of the indications for the use of G-CSF, taking into account not only the aggressiveness of the chemotherapy but also the characteristics of the patients.

Few trials have been conducted so far to elaborate clinical models using the patient's characteristics for predicting the risk of FN. However, such predictive factors exist and might more or less significantly influence the level of risk for FN. Patient-related predictive factors for FN that might be significant are indicated in Table 2.2 [29].

In a recent study in patients with hematological malignancies, an attempt has been made to incorporate some of these factors into a predictive model, namely the underlying disease, the involvement of the bone marrow, a body surface less than 2 m², a baseline monocyte lower than 150 µl, and the baseline hemoglobin level [2]. A rule of prediction of FN was computed with a sensitivity 78.6%, specificity 62.3%, positive predictive value 42.7%, and negative predictive value 89.1%.

A systematic review of the literature confirmed that age, performance status, and nutritional status are associated with a higher risk of FN [30] and various comorbid conditions, such as renal and liver function

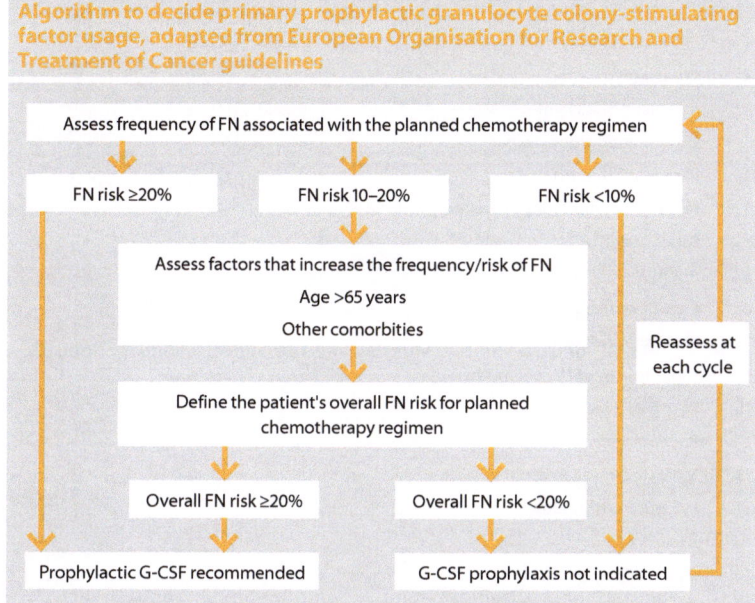

Figure 2.2 Algorithm to decide primary prophylactic granulocyte colony-stimulating factor usage, adapted from European Organisation for Research and Treatment of Cancer guidelines. FN, febrile neutropenia; G-CSF, granulocyte colony-stimulating factor. Reproduced with permission from © Pergamon 2013, Aapro et al [1]. All Rights Reserved.

impairment, heart disease, and hypertension as well as obstructive lung disease, are associated with more frequent complications during FN [1].

Although the aggressiveness of chemotherapy currently remains the main predictive factor for the risk of chemotherapy-associated FN (and thus for deciding whether or not primary prophylaxis with G-CSF is indicated), it is nonetheless clear that many other factors, namely age and major comorbidities, must influence the clinician's decision. Until reliable predictive tools are developed, the decision should be made on the basis of presently available clinical evidence and medical expertise.

Should the indications for primary prophylaxis with granulocyte colony-stimulating factor be extended?

There are actually several reasons that militate for the extension of the indications for primary prophylaxis with G-CSF (Table 2.3).

	Factors potentially associated with an increased risk for developing febrile neutropenia during chemotherapy
1.	Older age
2.	Advanced disease/metastases
3.	No antibiotic prophylaxis
4.	Prior febrile neutropenia
5.	No granulocyte colony-stimulating factor use
6.	Female sex
7.	Anemia
8.	Cardiovascular disease
9.	Abnormal liver tests
10.	High-dose intensity chemotherapy
11.	Poor performance status
12.	Poor nutrition
13.	More than one comorbidity
14.	Lymphoma histology
15.	Asian origin
16.	Body surface less than 2 m^2
17.	Pretreatment neutrophils less than 1.5
18.	Albumin less than 3.5 g/dl

Table 2.2 Factors potentially associated with an increased risk for developing febrile neutropenia during chemotherapy. Reproduced with permission from © Lippincott Williams & Wilkins 2013, Lyman, Shayne [29]. All Rights Reserved.

The prediction of the risk of FN based solely on the type of chemotherapy administered is not entirely reliable; in addition, elderly patients and those with various comorbidities have an increased risk of FN with a given chemotherapy regimen and present more frequently with complications if FN occurs.

Many regimens used for the treatment of patients with solid tumors have a risk of FN lower than 20%. On the other hand, when FN occurs in such patients, the morbidity and mortality that are associated with it are in the same range as what is observed in patients with a high risk of development of FN [31]. We have observed that FN, in patients with a <10% and <20% risk of developing FN, has a frequency of complications of 9% and 10% and a mortality of 4% and 6%, respectively. Moreover, it has been reported that in patients with a moderate risk of FN (<20%), impaired chemotherapy delivery (timing and dose) was

	Reasons for extending the indications for primary prophylaxis with granulocyte colony-stimulating factor to patients with a <20% risk of febrile neutropenia
1.	Type of chemotherapy does not accurately predict the risk of FN
2.	Older age and various comorbidities increase the risk of FN for a given chemotherapy regimen and increase the risk of complications resulting from FN
3.	Many common chemotherapy regimens are associated with <20% risk of FN; these patients are denied prophylaxis with G-CSF
4.	The frequency of complications and mortality associated with FN are the same regardless of the initial risk for FN
5.	Patients with a low risk of FN benefit from primary prophylaxis in terms of a reduced incidence of FN
6.	Cost effectiveness in patients with a low risk of developing FN during chemotherapy might be dealt with through reduced dosage of G-CSF and use of biosimilars

Table 2.3 Reasons for extending the indications for primary prophylaxis with granulocyte colony-stimulating factor to patients with a <20% risk of febrile neutropenia. FN, febrile neutropenia; G-CSF, granulocyte colony-stimulating factor.

observed in 40% of the patients developing FN [32]. Additionally, there is evidence that these patients, with a low or moderate risk of developing FN during chemotherapy administration, significantly benefit from primary prophylaxis with G-CSF [31,32].

Conversely, it was found that a lower baseline risk for FN might be associated with a greater reduction in the relative risk by G-CSF [18]. This can explain why noncontinuous G-CSF therapy may be safe in patients at a relatively low risk of FN, as suggested by Papaldo et al [33]; these investigators evaluated different G-CSF schedules in patients with breast cancer and an overall risk rate for FN of 7%; they found that 300 µg/day of filgrastim on days 8 and 12 were just as efficacious as more standard regimens (eg, days 8–14) or higher doses of G-CSF. These retrospective investigations are supported by more recent prospective studies [34], suggesting that shorter G-CSF schedules (eg, on days 5, 7, 9, 11) were more active than standard filgrastim or pegfilgrastim in patients with breast cancer receiving adjuvant dose-dense chemotherapy, with a 6% risk of FN (historical controls).

At the present time, these observations suggest that a large proportion of the patients receiving chemotherapy is left without protection against FN, just for economic reasons. As will be discussed later, the cost effectiveness of primary prophylaxis with G-CSF may improve by the rational use of reduced doses of G-CSF and utilization of less expensive biosimilars, leading to other paradigms for prophylaxis than those proposed today (Figure 2.3), although these proposals need prospective controlled validation.

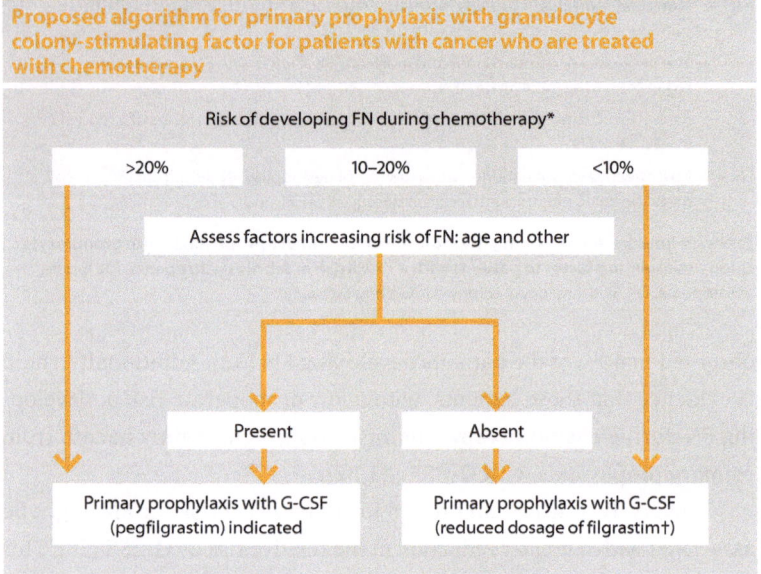

Figure 2.3 Proposed algorithm for primary prophylaxis with granulocyte colony-stimulating factor for patients with cancer who are treated with chemotherapy.
*Based on the aggressiveness of the regimen; †Use biosimilars if available. FN, febrile neutropenia; G-CSF, granulocyte colony-stimulating factor.

References

1   Aapro MS, Bohlius J, Cameron DA, et al; European Organisation for Research and Treatment of Cancer. 2010 update of EORTC guidelines for the use of granulocyte-colony stimulating factor to reduce the incidence of chemotherapy-induced febrile neutropenia in adult patients with lymphoproliferative disorders and solid tumours. *Eur J Cancer.* 2011;47:8-32.

2   Moreau M, Klastersky J, Schwartzbold A, et al. A general chemotherapy myelotoxicity score to predict febrile neutropenian hematological malignancies. *Ann Oncol.* 2009;20:513-519.

3   Hansson EK, Friberg LE. The shape of the myelosuppression time profile is related to the probability of developing neutropenic fever in patients with docetaxel-induced grade IV neutropenia. *Cancer Chemother Pharmacol.* 2012;69:881-890.

4   Chen C, Chan A, Yap K. Visualizing clinical predictors of febrile neutropenia in Asian cancer patients receiving myelosuppressive chemotherapy. *J Oncol Pharm Pract.* 2012;19:111-120.

5   Chang LL, Schneider SM, Chiang SC, Horng CF. Implementing an evidence-based risk assessment tool to predict chemotherapy-induced neutropenia in women with breast cancer. *Cancer Nurs.* 2013;36:198-205.

6   Klastersky J, Gombos A, Georgala A, Awada A. Prevention of neutropenia-related events in elderly patients with hematological cancer. *Aging Health.* 2011;7:829-842.

7   Bagnasco F, Haupt R, Fontana V, et al. Risk of repeated febrile episodes during chemotherapy-induced granulocytopenbia in children with cancer: a prospective center study. *J Chemother.* 2012;24:155-160.

8   Schlesinger A, Paul M, Gafter-Gvili A, Rubinovitch B, Leibovici L. Infection-control interventions for cancer patients after chemotherapy: a systematic review and meta-analysis. *Lancet Infect Dis.* 2009;9:97-107.

9   Klastersky J, Debusscher L, Weerts D, Daneau D. Use of oral antibiotics in protected units environment: clinical effectiveness and role in the emergence of antibiotic-resistant strains. *Pathol Biol (Paris).* 1974;22:5-12.

10 Trimethoprim-sulfamethoxazole in the prevention of infection in neutropenic patients. EORTC International Antimicrobial Therapy Project Group. *J Infect Dis.* 1984;150:372-379.

11 Gafter-Gvili A, Fraser A, Paul M, Leibovici L. Meta-analysis: antibiotic prophylaxis reduces mortality in neutropenic patients. *Ann Intern Med.* 2005;142:979-995.

12 Gafter-Gvili A, Paul M, Fraser A, Leibovici L. Effects of quinolone prophylaxis in afebrile neutropenic patients on microbial resistance. Systematic review and meta-analysis. *J Antimicrob Chemother.* 2007;59:5-22.

13 Smith T, Khatcheressian J, Lyman GH, et al. 2006 update of recommendations for the use of white blood cell growth factors: an evidence-based clinical practice guideline. *J Clin Oncol.* 2006;24:3187-3205.

14 Klastersky J, Paesmans M, Georgala A, et al. Outpatients oral antibiotics for febrile neutropenic cancer patients using a score predictive for complications. *J Clin Oncol.* 2006;24:4129-4134.

15 Sebban C, Dussart S, Fuhrmann C, et al. Oral moxiflacin or intravenous ceftriaxone for the treatment of low-risk neutropenic fever in cancer patients suitable for early hospital discharge. *Support Care Cancer.* 2008;16:1017-1023.

16 Laoprasopwattana K, Khwanna T, Suwankeeree P, Sujjanunt T, Tunyapanit W, Chelae S. Ciprofloxacin reduces occurrence of fever in children with acute leukemia who develop neutropenia during chemotherapy. *Pediatr Infect Dis J.* 2013;32:e94-e98.

17 Bron D. Bone Marrow Transplantation. In: Klastersky J, Schimpff SC, Senn HJ, eds. Supportive Care in Cancer, *A Handbook for Oncologists, Second Edition, Revised and Expanded.* New York, NY: Marcel Decker; 1999:166-185.

18 Kuderer NM, Dale DC, Crawford J, Lyman GH. Impact of primary prophylaxis with granulocyte colony-stimulating factor on febrile neutropenia and mortality in adult cancer patients receiving chemotherapy: a systematic review. *J Clin Oncol.* 2007;25:3158-3167.

19 Cooper KL, Madan J, Whyte S, Stevenson MD, Akehurst RL. Granulocyte colony-stimulating factors for febrile neutropenia prophylaxis following chemotherapy: systematic review and meta-analysis. *BMC Cancer.* 2011;11:404.

20 Sunhwa K, Baek J, Min H. Effects of prophylactic hematopoietic colony stimulating factors on stem cell transplantations: meta-analysis. *Arch Pharm Res.* 2012;35:2013-2020.

21 Aapro M, Crawford J, Kamioner D. Prophylaxis of chemotherapy-induced febrile neutropenia with granulocyte colony-stimulating factors: where are we now? *Support Care Cancer.* 2010;18:529-541.

22 Crawford J, Ozer H, Stoller R, et al. Reduction by granulocyte colony-stimulating factor of fever and neutropenia induced by chemotherapy in patients with small-cell lung cancer. *N Engl J Med.* 1991;325:164-170.

23 Lalami Y, Paesmans M, Aoun M, et al. A prospective randomized evaluation of G-CSF or G-CSF plus oral antibiotics in chemotherapy-treated patients at high risk of developing febrile neutropenia. *Support Care Cancer.* 2004;12:725-730.

24 Lyman GH, Morrison VA, Dale DC, Crawford J, Delgado DJ, Fridman M; OPPS Working Group; ANC Study Group. Risk of febrile neutropenia in patients with intermediate-grade non-Hodgkin's lymphoma receiving CHOP chemotherapy. *Leuk Lymphoma.* 2003;44:2069-2076.

25 Martín M, Lluch A, Seguí MA, et al. Toxicity and health-related quality of life in breast patients receiving adjuvant docetaxel, doxorubicin, cyclophosphamide (TAC) or 5-fluorouracil, doxorubicin and cyclophosphamide (FAC): impact of adding primary prophylactic granulocyte-colony stimulating factor to the TAC regimen. *Ann Oncol.* 2006;17:1205-1212.

26 Klastersky J, Awada A. Prevention of febrile neutropenia in chemotherapy-treated cancer patients: pegylated versus standard myeloid colony stimulating factors. Do we have a choice? *Crit Rev Oncol Hematol.* 2011;78:17-23.

27 Naeim A, Henk HJ, Becker L, et al. Pegfilgrastim prophylaxis is associated with a lower risk of hospitalization of cancer patients than filgrastim prophylaxis: a retrospective United States claims analysis of granulocyte colony-stimulating factors (G-CSF). *BMC Cancer.* 2013;3:11.

28 Ziakas PD, Kourbeti IS. Pegfilgrastim vs. filgrastim for supportive care after autologous stem cell transplantation: can we decide? *Clin Transplant.* 2012;26:16-22.

29 Lyman GH, Shayne M. Granulocyte colony-stimulating factors: finding the right indication. *Curr Opin Oncol.* 2007;19:299-307.

30 Wingard JR, Elmongy M. Strategies for minimizing neutropenic lever's complications: prophylactic myeloid growth factors or antibiotics. *Crit Rev Oncol Hematol.* 2009;72:144-154.

31 Klastersky J, Georgala A, Ameye L, et al. Febrile neutropenia occurring in patients with solid tumors: is the risk of complications affected by the type of chemotherapy? *Support Care Cancer.* 2010;18(Suppl 3):S101-S102.

32 Gerlier L, Lamotte M, Awada A, et al. The use of chemotherapy regimens carrying a moderate or high risk of febrile neutropenia and the corresponding management of febrile neutropenia: an expert survey in breast cancer and non-Hodgkin's lymphoma. *BMC Cancer.* 2010;10:642.

33 Papaldo P, Lopez M, Marolla P, et al. Impact of five prophylactic filgrastim schedules on hematologic toxicity in early breast cancer patients treated with epirubicin and cyclophosphamide. *J Clin Oncol.* 2005;23:6908-6918.

34 Hendler D, Shulamith R, Yerulshalmi, et al. Different schedules of granulocyte growth factor support for patients with breast cancer receiving adjuvant dose-dense chemotherapy. *Am J Clin Oncol.* 2011;34:619-624.

Chapter 3

Prediction of the risk of complications associated with febrile neutropenia

Types and incidence of complications

Febrile neutropenia (FN) is associated with a significant incidence of complications, the most serious of which are listed in Table 3.1 [1]. These complications occur in about 10% of patients with FN and are more frequent in patients with bacteremia (20%). In addition to these complications, which often require vigorous and prolonged therapy, there are indirect and less well-measurable consequences of FN, such as possible reduction of efficacy of chemotherapy through reduction of doses or delays of administration, psychosocial burden to the patient and their family as well as social and financial cost. Moreover, death occurs in about 3–4% of patients as a result of FN; the mortality is higher in patients with bacteremia (10%) [2].

While the presence of bacteremia is associated with a higher incidence of complications and higher mortality, it is not very helpful for clinical early prediction at the onset of FN to know whether bacteremia is present or not; in addition, the early diagnosis of bacteremia at the onset of FN is difficult [3].

The type of underlying neoplasia (hematological cancer or solid tumor) does not appear to influence the incidence of complications or mortality. However, since the time when FN was recognized as a major problem in patients with cancer [4,5], the exposed population to chemotherapy has considerably changed and the overall support to the patients has

J. A. Klastersky, *Febrile Neutropenia*,
DOI: 10.1007/978-1-907673-70-2_3, © Springer Healthcare 2014

Serious medical complications of febrile neutropenia
Hypotension: systolic blood pressure <90 mm Hg or need for pressure support to maintain blood pressure
Respiratory failure: arterial oxygen pressure <60 mm Hg while breathing room air or need for mechanical ventilation
Disseminated intravascular coagulation
Confusion or altered mental state
Congestive cardiac failure seen on chest x-ray and requiring treatment
Bleeding severe enough to require transfusion
Arrhythmia or electrocardiographic changes requiring treatment
Renal failure requiring investigation and/or treatment with intravenous fluids, dialysis, or any other intervention

Table 3.1 Serious medical complications of febrile neutropenia. Reproduced with permission from © American Society of Clinical Oncology 2013, Klastersky et al [1]. All Rights Reserved.

markedly improved; therefore, it was recognized that FN has become a heterogeneous syndrome with different outcomes in terms of vital prognosis and severity of various complications.

Prediction of the individual risk of complications

There have been several attempts to predict a low risk of complications in patients with FN, without achieving a general consensus. Among these early attempts, Talcott et al [6] proposed a model which considered low-risk outpatients at presentation, not requiring hospitalization for another reason than FN itself, and having adequately controlled cancer. Unfortunately, while that model was reliable for predicting patients with FN at low risk of complications, it was not effective for safely selecting low-risk patients for home therapy.

In a multinational, multicenter study of more than 1100 patients with FN, the study section on infection of the Multinational Association for Supportive Care in Cancer (MASCC) demonstrated that a series of characteristics, easily identifiable at the onset of FN, could reliably predict a low risk of complications. Using these factors, a simple and easy-to-use MASCC risk index has been developed (Table 3.2) [1,7]. Since then, this risk index has been widely accepted as a standard technique to evaluate the risk of complications in patients with FN, namely by European Society of Medical Oncology (ESMO) and Infectious Diseases Society of America (IDSA). The MASCC model has been validated in many studies [7]; the

Multinational Association of Supportive Cancer Care scoring system	
Characteristic	**Weight**
Burden of illness: no or mild symptoms	5
No hypotension	5
No chronic obstructive pulmonary disease	4
Solid tumor or no previous fungal infection	4
No dehydration	3
Burden of illness: moderate symptoms	3
Outpatient status	3
Age <60 years	2

Table 3.2 Multinational Association of Supportive Cancer Care scoring system. Points attributed to the variable "burden of illness" are not cumulative. The maximum theoretical score is therefore 26. Reproduced with permission from © Springer-Verlag 2013, Klastersky, Paesmans [7]. All Rights Reserved.

most recent validation in 227 prospectively enrolled patients showed a sensitivity, specificity, positive predictive value, and negative predictive value of 81%, 60%, 86%, and 52%, respectively.

Because the severity and duration of neutropenia [8] are not included in the MASCC model, there has been some concern about the value of the MASCC score index in patients with hematological malignancies. Recently, the MASCC score has been validated in patients with hematological malignancies [9,10], which indicated that the MASCC score index was indeed a useful predictor of outcome in those patients and was widely applicable.

The overall review of the studies that validated the MASCC score is indicated in Table 3.3 [7–14].

Laboratory data and the Multinational Association of Supportive Cancer Care score index

Although laboratory data (biomarkers or microbiological results) are usually not available to the clinician at the onset of fever and/or patient's presentation at the emergency department, various biological parameters have been evaluated as potentially useful markers of the risk of more severe infection in patients with FN. Among the biomarkers that have been evaluated, the most frequently studied are C-reactive protein (CRP), procalcitonin, neopterin, interleukin (IL)-6, and IL-8. Uys et al attempted to combine all these biological markers with the MASCC score

Reference	No. of episodes	Patients with hematological malignancy (%)	Predicted at low risk (%)	Se (%)	Sp (%)	PPV (%)	NPV (%)
Paesmans [7]	1003	55	72	79	56	88	40
Stratum of hematological tumors	549	100	70	77	51	84	40
Stratum of solid tumor patients	454	0	74	81	64	93	38
Uys et al [12]	80	30	73	95	95	98	86
Cherif et al [9]	279	100	38	59	87	85	64
Klastersky et al [14]	611	43	72	78	54	88	36
Innes et al [13]	100	6	90	92	40	97	20
Baskaran et al [10]	116	100	71	93	67	83	85
Pun Hui et al [8]	227	20	70	81	60	86	52
Carmona-Bayonas et al[11]*	169	0	?	94	36	NA	NA

Table 3.3 Studies validating the Multinational Association of Supportive Cancer Care score index. *Selected patients populations ("apparently" stable patients). The characteristics were calculated for a test aiming to identify low-risk patients and may then differ from the original publications. Due to the case-control design of the study, the rate of patients predicted at low risk as well as the negative and positive predictive values is meaningless. NPV, negative predictive value; PPV, positive predictive value; Se, sensitivity; Sp, specificity. Reproduced with permission from © Springer-Verlag 2013, Klastersky, Paesmans [7]. All Rights Reserved. Adapted from Pun Hui et al [8]; Cherif et al [9]; Baskaran et al [10]; Carmona-Bayonas et al [11]; Uys et al [12]; Innes et al [13]; Klastersky et al [14].

index [15]. Multivariate analysis revealed that the MASCC score, but none of the laboratory parameters, was an accurate and independent variable for prediction of resolution of FN, with or without complications or death. Of these various laboratory parameters, procalcitonin had the strongest association with the MASCC index. It was concluded that the MASCC score was a useful predictor of outcome while measurements of procalcitonin, CRP, IL-6, and IL-8 were of limited value.

However, others have found that CRP and IL-8 were predictors of sepsis, bacteremia, and severe complications, especially in children [16]. These observations suggest that there might be predictive factors for sepsis and its complications. These aspects will be discussed later.

The prediction of bacteremia is difficult and does not modify the predictive value of the MASCC index [3]. It is possible that it is not bacteremia by itself that carries a poor prognosis but some clinical manifestations associated with it and representing surrogates for development of severe complications, such as septic shock.

The predictive value of the Multinational Association of Supportive Cancer Care index

The MASCC scoring index system was initially designed to predict patients with FN who were at low risk of complications and death, with the implicit goal to have those patients benefit from simpler and perhaps less expensive therapies. Our MASCC model represents an improvement over the Talcott's classification as it has a lower misclassification rate (30% vs 59%) and a better sensitivity (63% vs 26%).

Rather than considering an "uncontrolled cancer" variable, the MASCC index uses factors more specifically associated with the clinical severity of FN (eg, burden of illness, hypotension, and dehydration). We attempted to replace "burden of illness" in our model with more specific criteria, but none of these attempts had been successful and burden of illness was kept as a pivotal aspect of the MASCC scoring system [7] for the prediction of patients with FN who are at low risk of complications.

A MASCC score ≥21 predicts a risk <5% of developing severe complications during an episode of FN [1]. In a recent validation of our model, it was found that 12% of the patients predicted at low risk (MASCC score ≤21) developed complications and 2% died; when using the Talcott's predictive rules, the authors found in the low-risk group a frequency of complications of 43% and a mortality of 9% [8]. Quite interestingly, the use of the MASCC score index proved to be also useful to predict which patients might be at a higher risk of complications and death during an episode of FN. In a large review of bacteremia in patients with FN, we found that while the overall rates of complications and death in the low-risk patients were 18% and 3%, respectively, the corresponding figures were 49% and 19% in patients with a MASCC score <21, a highly significant difference [2]. Further, when we stratified the patients with a low score, we found that patients with a score <15 had a much higher rate of complications compared to the outcome of patients with an intermediate score of 15–20. These observations are summarized in Table 3.4 [2].

Complications rate in patients with bacteremia stratified by classes of the Multinational Association of Supportive Cancer Care score and type of bacteremia (continues over)

MASCC Score	Single Gram-positive					Single Gram-negative				
	Total	Complications (non-lethal)		Death		Total	Complications (non-lethal)		Death	
<15	18	9	50%	5	28%	23	9	39%	10	43%
15–20	89	23	26%	5	6%	64	18	28%	15	23%
≥21	176	25	14%	3	2%	81	11	14%	5	6%

Table 3.4 Complications rate in patients with bacteremia stratified by classes of the Multinational Association of Supportive Cancer Care score and type of bacteremia (continues over).

Also, inpatients with both Gram-positive and Gram-negative bacteremia there is a significant difference in the frequency of overall complications and mortality between the patients with a MASCC score <21 or ≥21. We will come back to the MASCC score index to predict patients at high risk of developing complications during FN as well as other factors predictive of such complications, such as severe sepsis and septic shock (see page 46).

Currently, the MASCC score index has been adopted in international guidelines regarding the management of FN, namely the ESMO [17] and IDSA [18]. As indicated in Figure 3.1, it is now recommended to calculate the MASCC score when the patient steps into the hospital [17]. Patients predicted at low risk, might benefit from oral antimicrobial therapy and possibly outpatient management in some cases, at least. Patients predicted at a high risk should be hospitalized and rapidly treated with broad spectrum antibiotics administered intravenously. A particular attention should be paid to symptoms predictive of severe sepsis.

MASCC Score	Polymicrobial				
	Total	Complications (non-lethal)		Death	
<15	6	2		2	
15–20	9	2		2	
≥21	33	7	21%	2	6%

Table 3.4 Complications rate in patients with bacteremia stratified by classes of the Multinational Association of Supportive Cancer Care score and type of bacteremia (continued). The complications rate and death rate were only calculated in subgroups of more than 10 cases. MASCC, Multinational Association of Supportive Cancer Care. Reproduced with permission from © Elsevier 2013, Klastersky et al [2]. All Rights Reserved.

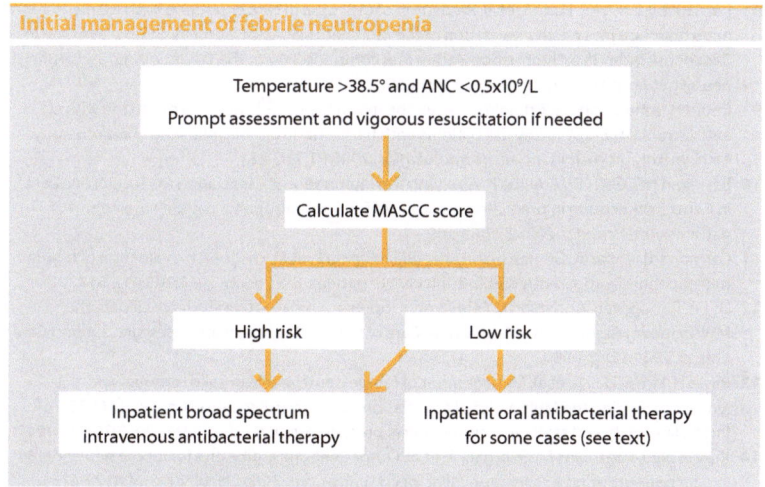

Figure 3.1 Initial management of febrile neutropenia. ANC, absolute neutrophil count; MASCC, Multinational Association of Supportive Cancer Care. Reproduced with permission from © Oxford University Press 2013, Marti et al [17]. All Rights Reserved.

References

1   Klastersky J, Paesmans M, Rubenstein EB, et al. The Multinational Association for Supportive Care in Cancer Risk Index: a multinational scoring system for identifying low-risk febrile neutropenic cancer patients. *J Clin Oncol.* 2000;18:3038-3051.

2   Klastersky J, Ameye L, Maertens J, et al. Bacteraemia in febrile neutropenic cancer patients. *Int J Antimicrob Agents.* 2007;30(Suppl 1):S51-S59.

3   Paesmans M, Klastersky J, Maertens J, et al. Predicting febrile neutropenic patients at low risk using the MASCC score: does bacteremia matter? *Support Care Cancer.* 2011;19:1001-1008.

4   McCabe WR, Jackson GG. Gram-negative bacteremia. *Int Arch Med.* 1962;110:92-100.

5   Bodey GP, Buckley M, Sathe Y, et al. Quantitative relationship between circulating leukocytes and infection in patients with acute leukemia. *Ann Intern Med.* 1996;64:328-340.

6   Talcott JA, Siegel RD, Finberg R, et al. Risk assessment in cancer patients with fever and neutropenia: a prospective, two-center validation of a prediction rule. *J Clin Oncol.* 1992;10:316-322.

7   Klastersky J, Paesmans M. The Multinational Association for Supportive Care in Cancer (MASCC) Risk Index: ten years of use identifying low-risk febrile neutropenic cancer patients. *Support Care Cancer.* 2013;21:1487-1495.

8   Pun Hui E, Leung KS, Poon T, et al. Prediction of outcome in cancer patients with febrile neutropenia: a prospective validation of the Multinational Association for Supportive Care in Cancer risk index in a Chinese population and comparison with the Talcott model and artificial neural network. *Support Care Cancer.* 2011;19:1625-1635.

9   Cherif H, Johansson E, Björkholm M, et al. The feasibility of early hospital discharge with oral antimicrobial therapy in low risk patients with febrile neutropenia following chemotherapy for hematologic malignancies. *Haematologica.* 2006;91:215-222.

10 Baskaran ND, Gan GG, Adeeba K. Applying the Multinational Association for Supportive Care in Cancer risk scoring in predicting outcome of febrile neutropenia patients in a cohort of patients. *Ann Hematol.* 2008;87:563-569.

11 Carmona-Bayonas A, Gómez J, González-Billalabeitia E, et al. Prognostic evaluation of febrile neutropaenia in apparently stable adult cancer patient. *Br J Cancer.* 2011;105:612-617.

12 Uys A, Rapoport B, Anderson R. Febrile neutropenia: a prospective study to validate the Multinational Association of Supportive Care of Cancer (MASCC) risk index score. *Support Care Cancer.* 2004;12:555-560.

13 Innes H, Lim S, Hall A, et al. Management of febrile neutropenia in solid tumours and lymphomas using the Multinational Association for Supportive Care in Cancer (MASCC) risk index: feasibility and safety in routine clinical practice. *Support Care Cancer.* 2008;16:485-4941.

14 Klastersky J, Paesmans M, Georgala A, et al. Outpatient oral antibiotics for febrile neutropenic cancer patients using a score predictive for complications. *J Clin Oncol.* 2006;24:4129-4134.

15 Uys A, Rapoport B, Meyer P, et al. Prediction of outcome in cancer patients with febrile neutropenia: comparison of the Multinational Association of Supportive Care in Cancer risk-index score with procalcitonin, C-reactive protein, serum amyloid A, and interleukins-1β, -6 and -10. *Eur J Cancer Care.* 2007;16:475-483.

16 Santolaya ME, Alvarez AM, Aviles CL, et al. Admission clinical and laboratory factors associated with death in children with cancer during a febrile neutropenic episode. *Pediatr Infect Dis J.* 2007;26:794-798.

17 Marti F, Cullen MH, Roila F. Management of febrile neutropenia: ESMO clinical recommendations. *Ann Oncol.* 2009;20:iv166-iv69.

18 Freifeld A, Bow E, Sepkowitz K, et al. Executive summary: clinical practice guideline for the use of antimicrobial agents in neutropenic patients with cancer: 2010 update by infectious diseases society of America. *Clin Infect Dis.* 2011;52:e56-e93.

Chapter 4

Management of the low-risk patients

Orally administered antimicrobial therapy

The Multinational Association of Supportive Cancer Care (MASCC) score index has been developed to predict a low risk (<5%) of complications in patients with febrile neutropenia (FN). In our original study, a score ≤21 identified low-risk patients with a positive predictive value of 91%, specificity of 68%, and sensitivity of 71% [1]; these patients had <5% of severe complications and 16% died (4 out of 243). More recent validations of the MASCC score have confirmed a somewhat higher frequency of complications (12–18%), but still a low mortality of 2–3% [2,3].

The paradigm of antimicrobial therapy for FN has been the intravenous administration broad spectrum antibiotics, either as combinations or single-drug therapy with extended spectrum agents [4]. This has been challenged by studies showing that in low-risk patients oral therapy with ciprofloxacin plus amoxicillin clavulanate was as effective as intravenous therapy [5]. More recently, oral moxifloxacin was demonstrated as efficacious as oral combination therapy in patients at low risk of infection during FN [6], which makes a schedule of a once daily administered oral antimicrobial therapy feasible [7].

Of course, there are limitations for the use of oral antimicrobial therapy; in a large study validating the concept of oral antibiotics for patients with FN and using the MASCC score for predicting a low risk of infection, we found that there were several reasons for not administering oral treatment to such patients [8]. As summarized in Table 4.1, these

J. A. Klastersky, *Febrile Neutropenia*,
DOI: 10.1007/978-1-907673-70-2_4, © Springer Healthcare 2014

Reasons for not administering oral treatment to patients predicted at low risk of serious complication development

Reason	No. of patients	%
Antibacterial prophylaxis and/or treatment	179	71
Inability to swallow	27	11
Contraindication(s) to oral therapy	17	6
Protocol violation	16	6
Refusal (by patient or physician)	11	5
Allergy to penicillin or quinolones	2	1

Table 4.1 Reasons for not administering oral treatment to patients predicted at low risk of serious complication development. Multinational Association for Supportive Care in Cancer score of ≥21. Reproduced with permission from © American Society of Clinical Oncology 2013, Klastersky et al [8]. All Rights Reserved.

were anterior antibacterial prophylaxis and/or treatment (71%), inability to swallow, other contraindications to oral therapy, refusal by the patient, or allergy to the proposed drugs [8]. In such cases, the intravenous administration of antibiotics is mandatory, although it does not preclude necessarily outpatient therapy [9].

On the other hand, the oral administration of antibiotics to patients with FN can be safely performed in hospitalized patients as shown in the initial studies testing the hypothesis of an effective oral antimicrobial therapy for low-risk patients with FN [5,10], with a potential for providing more comfort to the patients and for reducing the overall cost of management.

Fluoroquinolones have been the corner stone of orally administered antimicrobial therapy for low-risk patients with FN [5–7,10]. Of course, the major caveat with the use of fluoroquinolones for therapy is the potential emergence of resistant strains. The emergence of fluoroquinolone-resistant bacteria, namely *Escherichia coli*, in patients receiving fluoroquinolones as a prophylaxis for FN had been reported in the mid 1990s [11]; at that time, it was noted that these fluoroquinolone-resistant strains were also cross-resistant for all quinolones and multiresistant for a series of antibiotics, including trimethoprim-sulfamethoxazole, ampicillin, doxycycline, and others. The epidemiology of these fluoroquinolone-resistant *E. coli* can be altered by the antibiotic policy at a given center: a 6-month fluoroquinolone prophylaxis discontinuation decreased the incidence of resistant *E. coli* from >50% to 15%, but at the same time the incidence of Gram-negative bacteremia increased from 8% to 20%; the resumption of prophylaxis decreased the incidence of bacteremia and increased the frequency of resistant isolates to preintervention levels [12]. In another study on the epidemiological changes and emergence of resistance to fluoroquinolones in patients with hematological malignancies, 40% of those who were receiving prophylaxis with levofloxacin, isolation of resistant *E. coli* was independently associated with prophylaxis and duration (>7 days) of neutropenia [13]. In that study, there was a reduction of the incidence of FN with the use of levofloxacin prophylaxis and the infections caused by resistant strains did not show a worse outcome. However, in another study, patients with resistant strains (*E. coli* and *Klebsiella pneumoniae*) were significantly less likely to receive empirical therapy with activity against the offending pathogen, as a result of emergence of multiresistant bacteria [14]. The observation that these fluoroquinolone-resistant strains can be multiresistant is a major concern. For all these reasons, the extensive use of fluoroquinolones for prophylaxis of infection should be discouraged, as it reduces the availability of quinolones for oral therapy of FN [8], and more importantly might make these important antimicrobials globally useless.

Early hospital discharge

Although there are potential disadvantages with early hospital discharge (eg, the risk of noncompliance or limited supervision) for low-risk patients with FN, overall there are many positive aspects, including enhanced quality of life for the patients and lowered costs of care (Table 4.2) [15].

Innes et al [16] published a first prospective randomized comparative study between the standard approach (intravenous antibiotics in an inpatient setting) and a combination of oral therapy in outpatients. The latter approach was not inferior in terms of efficacy and resulted in an estimated 50% cost saving. In that study, the low-risk patients were selected using the Talcott's criteria with additional requirements for the sake of maximal safety, resulting in a very strict definition of "low risk" and thus limiting the eligible population. These authors, nonetheless, confirmed their initial observations in a subsequent study using the MASCC index

Advantages

- Avoidance of iatrogenic and other hazards of hospitalization
- Reduced rate of "healthcare associated" infections
- Lower cost of care
- Enhanced quality of life (patients)
- Increased convenience (family)
- More efficient resource utilization

Disadvantages

- Potential for serious complications in an unsupervised setting
- Potential for noncompliance
- Need to maintain an (expensive?) infrastructure

Table 4.2 Advantages and disadvantages of risk-based therapy outside of the hospital.
Reproduced with permission from © Taylor and Francis 2013, Rubinstein, Rolston [15].
All Rights Reserved.

score for selecting the low-risk patients [17], and validated its usefulness as a predictive score for a low risk of complications during FN.

Klastersky et al examined a similar strategy using the MASCC index score to define low risk in 611 consecutive patients with FN seen over 3 years at the Institut Jules Bordet [8]. Patients suitable for oral therapy with combination of amoxicillin clavulanate plus ciprofloxacin were eligible for discharge after a minimum 24-hour observation period. Eligible patients (n=178, 44%) were discharged within 2 days; no severe complications were observed and only 3 patients (4%) required readmission. The main reason for not administering oral antibiotics to otherwise low-risk patients was the concomitant use of antibacterial prophylaxis (71%); the main reason for prolonged hospitalization in patients eligible for early discharge was persistent fever, need for treatment change, or other medical complications during the 24-hour observation period; in those patients, the rate of severe medical complication was 9% (Table 4.3) [8].

In a similar study, Cherif et al confirmed the value of the MASCC score for identifying low-risk patients with hematological malignancies [18]. In that series, all patients were started on intravenous antibiotics as inpatients and were transferred to oral therapy if they remained clinically stable and defervesced. There were only 3 (5%) readmissions; the mean hospital stay was 6 days, clearly longer than in the two preceding

Reasons for prolonged hospitalization in predicted low-risk patients receiving oral empiric treatment

Reason	No. of patients
Persistent fever and need for treatment change	19
Objective medical reason	42
Subjective medical reason	10
Reason not related to a medical event	28

Table 4.3 Reasons for prolonged hospitalization in predicted low-risk patients receiving oral empiric treatment. Reproduced with permission from © American Society of Clinical Oncology 2013, Klastersky et al [8]. All Rights Reserved.

studies, which mostly included patients with solid tumors. A similar strategy of a prompt step-down from intravenous to oral therapy was found not inferior to full inpatient management with intravenous antibiotics in children with FN [19].

A meta-analysis of 10 studies comparing inpatient versus outpatient therapy of FN [20] did not find any significant difference in mortality or response rate. The readmission rate for the outpatient was 14% overall, primarily for persistent fever rather than life-threatening complications. That meta-analysis provides strong evidence that outpatient management of FN, in carefully selected patients, is as safe and effective as standard inpatient therapy.

More recently, Teuffel et al published another systematic review and meta-analysis of 14 randomized studies about outpatient management of cancer patients with FN [21]. They concluded that outpatient treatment of FN was a safe and efficacious alternative to inpatient management. The same group analyzed the cost effectiveness of outpatient treatment for FN in adult patients with cancer [22]; they concluded that, for such patients, hospital treatment is more expensive than outpatient strategies. A retrospective study by Elting et al also concluded that outpatient management of low-risk patients with FN was as safe and effective as inpatient management and significantly less costly [23].

Predicting the risk of serious complications during an episode of FN (by using validated tools, such as the MASCC index score) and predicting the safe early discharge from the hospital of a patient with FN on oral antimicrobial therapy remain somewhat different issues. In our study [8], we found that 9% of the patients who were not sent home after a 24-hour observation within the hospital developed serious complications, despite having been selected as low-risk patients by the MASCC scoring index at the time of their admission. The in-hospital observation is probably very important when selecting those patients suitable for early discharge. Nonetheless, many centers will send low-risk patients back home after a mere 4- to 8-hour observation period, after safely administering the first dose of prescribed antibiotics.

The most crucial approach for most of these patients is further, close monitoring. Patients should be given specific instructions if they feel worse or develop serious symptoms; they should be instructed to immediately seek medical advice or, even better, to return to the hospital. They should be encouraged to record their body temperature several times a day and to list their potential problems.

Those patients should be seen at follow-up clinics regularly and in between (contacted by phone) to review clinical and laboratory data and to make decisions regarding possible response failure, drug toxicity, and other potentially adverse events [24].

Table 4.4 summarizes the issues which will need more research to make orally administered regimens and early discharge for low-risk cancer patients with FN widely acceptable.

It is also possible that information on patients' preferences for out-patient treatment might help to optimize healthcare delivery to low-risk patients with FN. In a recent study [25], the probability of return to the hospital was the most important attribute to patients when considering home-based care for FN.

Remaining issues about the acceptance of orally administered antibiotics and early discharge for low-risk cancer patients with febrile neutropenia
Predictive factors for discharge
Standardized surveillance system
Education of physician and patient anxiety about safety
Demonstration of a quality-of-life benefit
Applicability to low income countries and rural areas
Definition of the cost effectiveness
Patients' preferences

Table 4.4 Remaining issues about the acceptance of orally administered antibiotics and early discharge for low-risk cancer patients with febrile neutropenia.

References

1   Klastersky J, Paesmans M, Rubenstein EB, et al. The Multinational Association for Supportive Care in Cancer Risk Index: a multinational scoring system for identifying low-risk febrile neutropenic cancer patients. *J Clin Oncol.* 2000;18:3038-3051.

2   Pun Hui E, Leung KS, Poon T, et al. Prediction of outcome in cancer patients with febrile neutropenia: a prospective validation of the Multinational Association for Supportive Care in Cancer risk index in a Chinese population and comparison with the Talcott model and artificial neural network. *Support Care Cancer.* 2011;19:1625-1635.

3   Klastersky J, Ameye L, Maertens, et al. Bacteraemia in febrile neutropenic cancer patients. *Int J Antimicrob Agents.* 2007;30(Suppl 1):S51-S59.

4   Paul M, Soares-Weiser K, Leibovici L. Beta lactam monotherapy versus beta lactam-aminoglycoside combination therapy for fever with neutropenia: systematic review and meta-analysis. *BMJ.* 2003;326:1111.

5   Kern WV, Cometta A, De Bock R, Langenaeken J, Paesmans M, Gaya H. Oral versus intravenous empirical antimicrobial therapy for fever in patients with granulocytopenia who are receiving cancer chemotherapy. International Antimicrobial Therapy Cooperative Group of the European Organization for Research and Treatment of Cancer. *N Engl J Med.* 1999;314:312-318.

6   Rolston KV, Frisbee-Hume SE, Patel S, Manzullo EF, Benjamin RS. Oral moxifloxacin for outpatients treatment of low-risk, febrile neutropenic patients. *Support Care Cancer.* 2010;18:89-94.

7   Kern WV, Marchetti O, Drgoina L, et al. Oral antibiotics for fever in low-risk neutropenic patients with cancer: a double-blind, randomized, multicenter trial comparing single daily moxifloxacin with twice daily ciprofloxacin plus amoxicillin/clavulanic acid combination therapy--EORTC infectious diseases group trial XV. *J Clin Oncol.* 2013;31:1149-1156.

8   Klastersky J, Paesmans M, Georgala A, et al. Outpatient oral antibiotics for febrile neutropenic cancer patients using a score predictive for complications. *J Clin Oncol.* 2006;24:4129-4134.

9   Talcott JA, Whalen A, Clark J, Rieker PP, Finberg R. Home antibiotic-therapy for low-risk cancer patients with fever and neutropenia-a pilot-study of 30 patients based on a validated prediction rule. *J Clin Oncol.* 1994;12:107-114.

10 Freifeld A, Marchigiani D, Walsh T, et al. A double blind comparison of empirical oral and intravenous antibiotic therapy for low-risk febrile patients with neutropenia during cancer chemotherapy. *N Engl J Med.* 1999;341:305-311.

11 Kern WV, Andriof E, Oethinger M, Kern P, Hacker J, Marre R. Emergence of fluoroquinolone-resistant Escherichia coli at a cancer center. *Antimicrob Agents Chemother.* 1994;38:681-687.

12 Kern WV, Klose K, Jellen-Ritter AS, et al. Fluoroquinolone resistance of Escherichia coli at a cancer center: epidemiologic evolution and effects of discontinuing prophylactic fluoroquinolone use in neutropenic patients with leukemia. *Eur J Clin Microbiol Infect Dis.* 2005;24:111-118.

13 Cattaneo C, Quaresmini G, Casari S, et al. Recent changes in bacterial epidemiology and the emergence of fluoroquinolone-resistant Escherichia coli among patients with haematological malignancies: results of a prospective study on 823 patients at a single institution. *J Antimicrob Chemother.* 2008;61:721-728.

14 Lautenbach E, Metlay JP, Bilker WB, Edelstein PH, Fishman NO. Association between fluoroquinolone resistance and mortality in Escherichia coli and Klebsiella pneumoniae infection: the role of inadequate empirical antimicrobial therapy. *Clin Infect Dis.* 2005;41:923-929.

15 Rubenstein EB, Rolston K VI. Risk-adjusted management of the febrile neutropenic cancer patient. In: Rolston RV, Rubinstein EB, eds *Textbook of Febrile Neutropenia.* London, UK: Martin Dunitz, Ltd; 2001:167-188.

16 Innes HE, Smith DB, O'Reilly SM, Clark PI, Kelly V, Marshall E. Oral antibiotics with early hospital discharge compared with in-patients intravenous antibiotics for low-risk febrile neutropenia in patients with cancer: a prospective randomized controlled single centre study. *Br J Cancer.* 2003;89:43-49.

17 Innes H, Lim SL, Hall A, Chan SY, Bhalla N, Marshall E. Management of febrile neutropenia in solid tumours and lymphomas using the Multinational Association for Supportive Care in Cancer (MASCC) risk index: feasibility and safety in routine clinical practice. *Support Care Cancer.* 2008;16:485-491.

18 Cherif H, Johansson E, Björkholm M, Kalin M. The feasibility of early hospital discharge with oral antimicrobial therapy in low risk patients with febrile neutropenia following chemotherapy for hematologic malignancies. *Haematologica.* 2006;91:215-222.

19 Brack E, Bodmer N, Simon A, et al. First-day step-down to oral outpatient treatment versus continued standard treatment in children with cancer and low-risk fever in neutropenia. A randomized controlled trial within the multicenter SPOG 2003 FN Study. *Pediatr Blood Cancer.* 2012;59:423-430.

20 Carstensen M, Sørensen JB. Outpatient management of febrile neutropenia: time to revise the present treatment strategy. *J Support Oncol.* 2008;6:199-208.

21 Teuffel O, Ethier MC, Alibhai SM, Beyene J, Sung L. Outpatient management of cancer patients with febrile neutropenia: a systematic review and meta-analysis. *Ann Oncol.* 2011;22:2358-2365.

22 Teuffel O, Amir E, Alibhai S, Beyene J, Sung L. Cost effectiveness of outpatient treatment for febrile neutropaenia in adult cancer patients. *Br J Cancer.* 2011;104:1377-1383.

23 Elting L, Lu C, Escalante C, et al. Outcomes and cost of outpatient or inpatient management of 712 patients with febrile neutropenia. *J Clin Oncol.* 2008;26:606-611.

24 Sebban C, Dussart S, Fuhrmann C, et al. Oral moxifloxacin or intravenous ceftriaxone for the treatment of low-risk neutropenic fever in cancer patients suitable for early hospital discharge. *Support Care Cancer.* 2008;16:1017-1023.

25 Lathia N, Isogai PK, Walker SE, et al. Eliciting patients' preferences for outpatient treatment of febrile neutropenia: a discrete choice experiment. *Support Care Cancer.* 2012;21:245-251.

Chapter 5

Management of the non-low-risk patients with febrile neutropenia

Predicting the non-low-risk patients with febrile neutropenia

In a large study combining the data from two sequential observational studies carried out by the Multinational Association for Supportive Care in Cancer (MASCC) Infection and Myelosuppression Study Group, we found that if the MASCC score was <21, the rates of complications and mortality was superior than in patients with a score ≥21 [1]. Moreover, as illustrated in Table 5.1, if the score was <15, serious complications (79%) and mortality (36%) were much higher; a score of 15–20 was indicative of an intermediate risk (40% and 14%, respectively, for complications and mortality) [1]. The use of the MASCC score for predicting patients

Risk-index score levels	Resolution without complications	Deaths
7–14 (*n*=33)	9 (27%)	8 (24%)
15–16 (*n*=38)	21 (55%)	7 (19%)
17–18 (*n*=58)	39 (67%)	8 (14%)
19–20 (*n*=90)	61 (68%)	9 (10%)
Total	130	32

Table 5.1 Clinical outcome of the patients not predicted as low risk by the Multinational Association for Supportive Care in Cancer risk score. $p<0.01$. Reproduced with permission from © Elsevier 2013, Klastersky et al [1]. All Rights Reserved.

J. A. Klastersky, *Febrile Neutropenia*,
DOI: 10.1007/978-1-907673-70-2_5, © Springer Healthcare 2014

with febrile neutropenia (FN) and a high risk of complications were also established by Blot and Nitenberg [2]; they suggested improving its performance by a repeated calculation of the severity score and by the inclusion of organ dysfunction. Nonetheless, no practical model was proposed. Another study by Ahn et al [3] confirmed the value of the MASCC score to predict poor outcome in patients with FN; in addition, they found that thrombocytopenia and increased C-reactive protein (CRP) were strongly associated with a poor prognosis.

Use of biological or microbiological parameters to predict poor outcome

An early study by Uys et al [4] did not find measurement of procalcitonin, CRP, and various interleukin (IL) to be helpful to increase the predictive value of the MASCC score. However, Ahn et al [3] found that thrombocytopenia and elevated CRP were strongly associated with a poor outcome, and similar conclusions were reported with IL-10 and procalcitonin as early predictors of complications in hematological patients with FN [5,6]. Although there is an interest for various laboratory markers (such as mannose-binding lectin, IL-6, IL-8, procalcitonin, and CRP) to be early markers of bacteremia in cancer patients with FN, no convincing evidence of their utility has been provided so far. Other approaches have used new biomarkers, such as pentraxin [7], for early detection of bacteremia. It was also suggested that the measurement of serum lactate in patients with FN might provide significant information about the risk of developing septic shock [8].

The presence of bacteremia in patients with FN increases the risk of severe complications and it is associated with higher mortality rates [1]. Although it has been shown that the diagnosis of bacteremia would not increase the power of predictability of the MASCC score in low-risk patients, it is unclear whether this is true in non-low-risk patients. In any case, the clinical diagnosis of bacteremia is difficult at the time of onset of FN, although it can be helped by the various technological improvements, such as the multiplex blood using polymerase chain reaction (PCR) amplification and DNA microarray hybridization [9,10], or other molecular approaches. Unfortunately, these laboratory data are not available readily when the patients come in, and under optimal conditions, they would be available with substantial delays. Thus, there is a need for prospective studies in non-low-risk patients using the MASCC score in addition to various biological and microbiological parameters to better predict the outcome of patients with FN.

Antibiotic management of non-low-risk patients

Non-low-risk patients with FN are commonly recommended to be treated with intravenously administered broad spectrum antibiotics. This approach is derived from the early experience of treating FN in patients with leukemia. In earlier studies, synergistic combinations of antibiotics were preferred as the response rate appeared significantly better than those obtained with single antibiotic treatment [11]. The beta-lactams and antipseudomonal aminoglycosides resulted in overall responses rates of 60–70%, a major progress indeed [12]. This type of combination for empirical therapy of FN is still popular, as shown in recent studies [13], but there is not convincing evidence that one broad-spectrum regimen is superior to another if the patterns of antimicrobial resistance are taken into account [14]. Actually, a systematic review and meta-analysis showed that there was no clinical advantage in treatment of FN with beta-lactam-aminoside combinations compared to broad spectrum beta-lactams as monotherapy [15], although that conclusion was less clear in high-risk patients. It should also be stressed that adverse events were significantly more common with the combination therapy, therefore, with the possible exception of high-risk patients, monotherapy for FN has become accepted as a paradigm.

A glycopeptide (vancomycin) is generally not given initially to patients with FN unless there is compelling evidence that Gram-positive infection is likely (eg, infected wound or intravenous catheter site, extensive mucositis) and in institutions having a high rate of infection with methicillin-resistant staphylococci.

Otherwise, the initial treatment (empiric therapy) should consist of a broad spectrum agent with activity against Gram-positive and Gram-negative common pathogens. Presently, ceftazidime, cefepime, piperacillin-tazobactam, imipenem, and meropenem are probably equally effective [16]. The actual choice in a given institution should be based on the local resistance patterns and the local overall antibiotic strategy. Several antimicrobial stewardship strategies, such as antimicrobial restriction, cycling, prospective audit, and feedback as well as de-escalation, have been evaluated in patients with cancer with a primary focus on the prevention and treatment of bacterial infections in patients with FN [17].

Non-low-risk patients at particular risk of septic complications

There are indications that the non-low-risk population might be heterogeneous; however, this has not been investigated yet in large adequately designed prospective trials. First, there is a strong correlation between the MASCC score level and the rate of complications or death (most often related to sepsis) in patients with FN (see Table 5.1); indeed, patients with bacteremia have a very high mortality rate if the MASCC score is <15, even for Gram-positive infections (28%, while 43% in patients with Gram-negative infections) [1] Another factor which may increase the rate of complications in cancer patients with bacteremia is the presence of a clinical focus of infection; Elting et al [18] observed a major difference in outcome between simple and complex infections in patients with FN.

Ahn et al [3] recently confirmed the value of the MASCC score to predict poor outcome in patients with FN; in addition, they found that thrombocytopenia and increased CRP were strongly associated with a poor prognosis. In that large series of 396 episodes of FN, there was an 18% incidence of severe complications and 4% of the patients died; these complications and deaths were associated overwhelmingly with sepsis.

It has also been reported that elevation of serum lactate at the time of FN in hemodynamically stable patients is strongly associated with the development of septic shock within 48 hours [19]. In addition, there have been several other recent attempts to predict septic complications in patients with FN, especially in patients with hematological malignancies [20–22].

How should these factors, predictive of septic complications in patients with FN, influence clinicians' decisions regarding the choice of initial antimicrobial therapy? An older, but essential study by the European

Organisation for Research and Treatment of Cancer (EORTC) demonstrated that combination therapy was associated with a better response rate to antimicrobial therapy in patients with severe (<100 granulocytes/cu mm) and persistent (<10 days) granulocytopenia [23]. The role of severity and duration of neutropenia has been clearly established in the earliest studies of FN [24] and should probably influence our decision for therapy. We will come back to these issues again with the problem of fungal infections (see page 56). The poor prognosis factors (Table 5.2) have not been adequately studied in specifically designed prospective trials and the available meta-analyses [15] do not properly answer the question of combination therapy in this subset of "poor-risk" patients. This has been actually recognized in the European Society of Medical Oncology (ESMO) Clinical Recommendations pertaining to the management of FN.

Based on the preceding considerations, it would seem sensible to expand the spectrum of the initial antimicrobial therapy for FN in those patients with a high risk of developing septic complications (Table 5.2). These patients should probably receive combination therapy with an antipseudomonal beta-lactam or penem and an aminoglycoside, combined or not to a glycopeptide, depending on the clinical presentation and the local epidemiological situation. Such combination regimens might provide the benefit of synergistic action and reduce the risk of not treating possible resistant strains. For the sake of safety, the combination should be adapted and de-escalated as soon as credible bacteriological data are available. It is also recognized that antimicrobial therapy might

Factors possibly predictive of severe sepsis and poor outcome in patients with febrile neutropenia
Multinational Association for Supportive Care in Cancer score <21
Thrombocytopenia (<10,000)
C-reactive protein ↗
Serum lactate ↗
Shock at presentation
Initial temperature <40°C
Granulocyte count <100
Clinical site of infection present

Table 5.2 Factors possibly predictive of severe sepsis and poor outcome in patients with febrile neutropenia.

not be the only parameter that influences the outcome of patients with FN and a high risk of developing septic complications.

Additional measures to possibly improve the outcome of patients with febrile neutropenia at high risk of septic complications

One of the arguably most important progresses that have been made in the management of FN is the wide acceptance for early empiric antimicrobial therapy [25]. The concept was formulated by Schimpff et al [12] based on the seminal observations of Bodey et al [24]. The concept has never been tested in a controlled trial, but its wide acceptance is the result of the improvement observed in the survival of FN once empiric therapy was applied [26,27]. In the earliest days of patients with FN evaluation, 50% of the patients with *Pseudomonas aeruginosa* or *Escherichia coli* sepsis were dead within 48 hours after drawing of the first blood culture.

Latency of the first dose of antibiotics (in addition to pneumonia and platelets counts of <50.000/cu mm) was identified as an independent factor associated with serious complications of FN [28]. Actually, the optimal time to administer antibiotics to a patient presenting to the emergency department with FN should be less than 60 minutes [25,29]; however, this is not always the case [30]. Although such a suboptimal timing before administration of therapy to patients with FN has been described in well-developed countries, the situation is probably much worse in countries with overall lower socioeconomic status [31,32].

Helpful evidence-based order sets to potentially improve initial antibiotic time intervals in patients with FN include [33]:

• staff education,
• placement of order-set antibiotics in unit-based dispensing machines, and
• intensive implication of the nursing staff.

These recommendations are probably valid for all patients with FN but could be life-saving in those with a high risk of development of severe sepsis. Thus, it is essential for non-low-risk patients with FN not to lose the "golden hour" for initiating antimicrobial therapy. Moreover, in those patients predicted at a high risk of developing septic shock, it might be wise to admit such patients into intensive care to provide them with the opportunity of close surveillance and early hemodynamic therapy if indicated [34].

As FN is by definition associated with neutropenia, which plays a major role in its pathogenesis, it may be asked whether rapid correction of neutropenia through the use of granulocyte transfusion or granulocyte colony-stimulating factor (G-CSF) might not be a sensible approach to the management of FN, especially in those patients with a predicted high risk of development of complications. Most clinical guidelines discourage the general use of G-CSF for adjunctive treatment of ongoing FN; however, its use in special situations, such as high risk for infectious complications, might be advised [35]. As far as granulocyte transfusions – a complicated and cumbersome procedure – are concerned, the concept has not gained wide acceptance perhaps because the majority of the studies were conducted before the era of G-CSFs [36]. Since then, small series continue to claim benefit from granulocyte transfusion in selected groups of patients [37].

Predictive factors of severe sepsis in patients with FN have not been adequately validated so far [38,39]; however, those patients who are predicted at a high risk of complications and/or sepsis on the basis of available evidence (Table 5.2) should promptly receive broad spectrum antimicrobial therapy, although this will not prevent the poor/fatal outcome in many of those patients. The issues of synergistic antimicrobial therapy, early intensive care management, and/or granulocyte transfusions can only be answered by adequately designed prospective trials.

Follow-up and assessment of response

The frequency of clinical assessment is determined by the severity of the course, but should be relatively high until the patient becomes afebrile and/or the granulocyte count clearly increases. This supervision of the patients is extremely important for those who are sent back home on orally administered antimicrobials and should be adequately organized through telephone calls, recurrent clinic visits, and close contacts with primary care physicians.

For patients who become afebrile after 48 hours and in whom the granulocyte count is $\geq 500 \times mm^3$, simplification of therapy can probably be made in most cases (eg, oral therapy, de-escalation from combination-to-single drug therapy, early discharge), especially in patients predicted at a low risk of complications.

For patients who are still febrile after 48 hours, clinical assessment of stability is essential. For stable patients, initial therapy should be continued for 24–48 hours and another reassessment should be made then.

For patients who are clinically deteriorating on initial empiric therapy, adjustment of antimicrobial therapy should be made on the basis of available microbiological evidence and clinical status. The advice of an infectious disease specialist should be requested and the admission to the intensive care unit should be considered. Special attention should be paid to the presence of factors predictive of severe sepsis and/or septic shock (Table 5.2).

Long-lasting fever for >4–6 days, even if the clinical deterioration is not obvious, should lead to the suspicion of occult fungal infection.

There are no strict rules about the duration of therapy in responding patients; if the patient is afebrile and the neutrophil count >500 × cu mm for 48 hours, therapy can be discontinued safely in most cases. In patients who are still neutropenic while having responded to initial therapy and are clinically stable for several days (5–7 days), therapy can be discontinued in most cases; these patients should be followed closely and the administration of G-CSF should be considered to speed up the granulocyte recovery.

The ESMO Clinical Recommendations for the management of FN [26] provide a sensible guideline for these situations (Figure 5.1) as well as the guidelines provided by the American Society of Clinical Oncology (ASCO) [40].

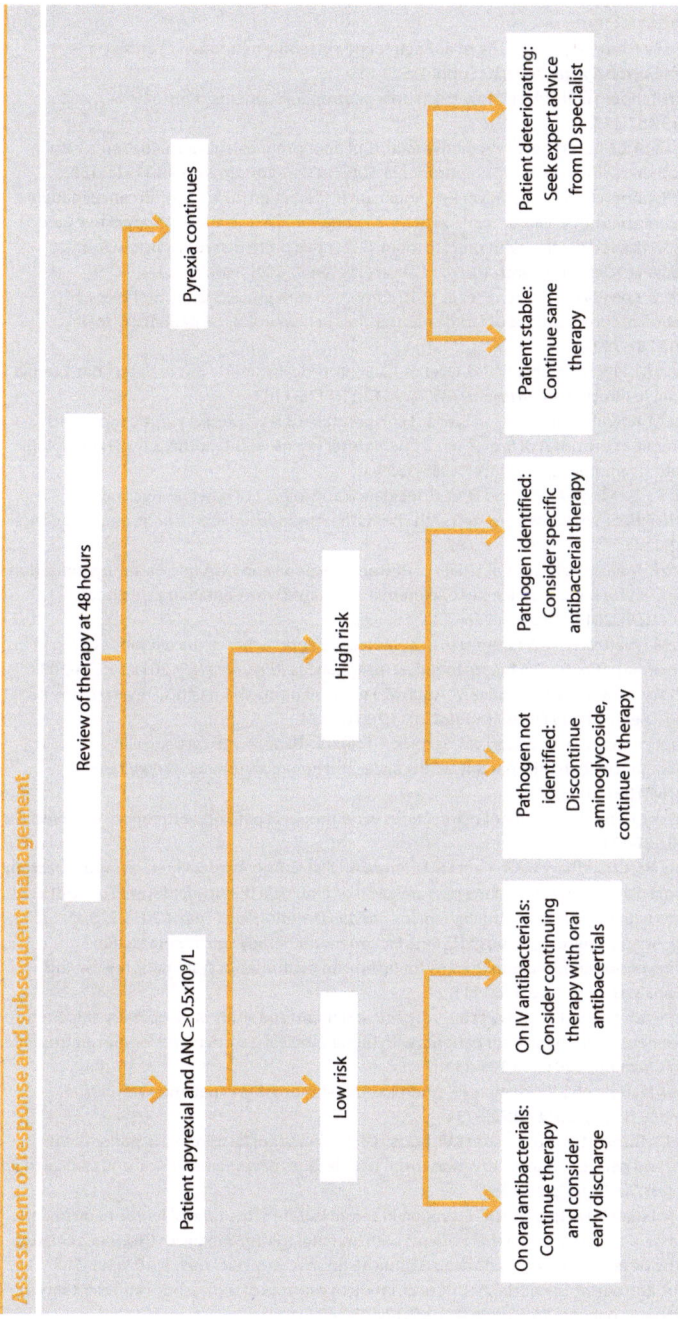

Figure 5.1 Assessment of response and subsequent management. ANC, absolute neutrophil count; ID, infectious disease; IV, intravenous. Reproduced with permission from © Oxford University Press 2013, Marti et al [26]. All Rights Reserved.

References

1   Klastersky J, Ameye L, Maertens, et al. Bacteraemia in febrile neutropenic cancer patients. *Int J Antimicrob Agents.* 2007;30(Suppl 1):S51-S59.

2   Blot F, Nitenberg G. [High and low-risk febrile neutropenic patients]. *Presse Med.* 2004;33:467-473.

3   Ahn S, Lee YS, Chun YH, et al. Predictive factors of poor prognosis in cancer patients with chemotherapy-induced febrile neutropenia. *Support Care Cancer.* 2011;19:1151-1158.

4   Uys A, Rapoport BL, Fickl H, Meyer PW, Anderson R. Prediction of outcome in cancer patients with febrile neutropenia: comparison of the Multinational Association of Supportive Care in Cancer risk-index score with procalcitonin, C-reactive protein, serum amyloid A, and interleukins-1beta, -6, -8 and -10. *Eur J Cancer Care (Engl).* 2007;16:475-483.

5   Vänskä M, Koivula I, Jantunen E, et al. IL-10 combined with procalcitonin improves early prediction of complications of febrile neutropenia in hematological patients. *Cytokine.* 2012;60:787-792.

6   Reitman AJ, Pisk RM, Gates JV 3rd, Ozeran JD. Serial procalcitonin levels to detect bacteremia in febrile neutropenia. *Clin Pediatr (Phila).* 2012;51:1175-1183.

7   Vänskä M, Koivula I, Hämäläinen S, et al. High pentraxin 3 level predicts septic shock and bacteremia at the onset of febrile neutropenia after intensive chemotherapy of hematologic patients. *Haematologica.* 2011;96:1385-1389.

8   Shaikh AJ, Bawany SA, Masood N, et al. Incidence and impact of baseline electrolyte abnormalities in patients admitted with chemotherapy induced febrile neutropenia. *J Cancer.* 2011;2:62-66.

9   Negoro E, Iwasaki H, Tai K, et al. Utility of PCR amplification and DNA microarray hybridization of 16S rDNA for rapid diagnosis of bacteremia associated with hematological diseases. *Int J Infect Dis.* 2013;17:e271-e276.

10 Guido M, Quattrocchi AZ, Pasanisi G, et al. Molecular approaches of the diagnosis of sepsis in neutropenic patients with haematological malignancies. *J Prev Med Hyg.* 2012;53:104-108.

11 Klastersky J, Awada A, Paesmans M, Aoun M. Febrile neutropenia: a critical review of the initial management. *Crit Rev Oncol Hematol.* 2011;78:185-194.

12 Schimpff S, Satterlee W, Young VM, Serpick A. Empiric therapy with carbenicillin and gentamicin for febrile patients with cancer and granulocytopenia. *N Engl J Med.* 1971;284:1061-1065.

13 Klastersky J. Empiric treatment of infections in neutropenic patients with cancer. *Rev Infect Dis.* 1983;5:S21-S31.

14 Ghalaut PS, Chaudhary U, Ghalaut VS, Dhingra A, Dixit G, Aggarwal S. Piperacillin-tazobactum plus amikacin versus ceftazidime plus amikacin as empirical therapy for fever in neutropenic patients with hematological malignancies. *Indian J Hematol Blood Transf.* 2011;27:131-135.

15 Paul M, Soares-Weiser K, Leibovici L. Beta lactam monotherapy versus beta lactam-aminoglycoside combination therapy for fever with neutropenia: systematic review and meta-analysis. *BMJ.* 2003;326:1111.

16 Nakagawa Y, Suzuki K, Ohta K, et al. Prospective randomized study of cefepime, panipenem, or meropenem monotherapy for patients with hematological disorders and febrile neutropenia. *J Infect Chemother.* 2013;19:103-111.

17 Tverdek FP, Rolston KV, Chemaly RF. Antimicrobial stewardship in patients with cancer. *Pharmacotherapy.* 2012;32:722-734.

18 Elting LS, Rubenstein EB, Rolston KVI, Bodey GP. Outcomes of bacteremia in patients with cancer and neutropenia: observations from two decades of epidemiological and clinical trials. *Clin Infect Dis.* 1997;25:247-259.

19 Mato A, Luger S, Heitjan D, et al. Elevation in serum lactate at the time of febrile neutropenia (FN) in hemodynamically-stable patients with hematologic malignancies (HM) is associated with the development of septic shock within 48 hours. *Cancer Biol Ther.* 2010;9:585-589.

20 Jeddi R, Zarrouk M, Benabdennebi Y, et al. Predictive factors of septic shock and mortality in neutropenic patients. *Hematology.* 2007;12:543-548.

21 Nakagawa Y, Suzuki K, Masaoka T. Evaluation of the risk factors for febrile neutropenia associated with hematological malignancy. *J Infect Chemother.* 2009;15:174-179.

22 Park Y, Kim D, Park S, et al. The suggestion of a risk stratification system for febrile neutropenia in patients with hematologic disease. *Leuk Res.* 2010;34:294-300.

23 Ceftazidime combined with a short or long course of amikacin for empirical therapy of gram-negative bacteremia in cancer patients with granulocytopenia. The EORTC International Antimicrobial Therapy Cooperative Group. *N Engl J Med.* 1978;317:1692-1698.

24 Bodey GP, Buckley M, Sathe YS, Freireich EJ. Quantitative relationship between circulating leukocytes and infection in patients with acute leukemia. *Ann Intern Med.* 1966;64:328-340.

25 Burry E, Punnett A, Mehta A, et al. Identification of educational and infrastructural barriers to prompt antibiotic delivery in febrile neutropenia: a quality improvement initiative. *Pediatr Blood Cancer.* 2012;59:431-435.

26 Marti FM, Cullen MH, Roila F; ESMO Guidelines Working Group. Management of febrile neutropenia: ESMO clinical recommendations. *Ann Oncol.* 2009;20:66-69.

27 Klastersky J. The changing face of febrile neutropenia-from monotherapy to moulds to mucositis. Why empirical therapy? *J Antimicrob Chemother.* 2009;63(Suppl 1):i14-i15.

28 Lynn JJ, Chen KF, Weng YM, Chiu TF. Risk factors associated with complications in patients with chemotherapy-induced febrile neutropenia in emergency department. *Hematol Oncol.* 2013 Jan 9. [Epub ahead of print].

29 Volpe D, Harrison S, Damian F, et al. Improving timeliness of antibiotic delivery for patients with fever and suspected neutropenia in a pediatric emergency department. *Pediatrics.* 2012;130:e201-e210.

30 Sammut SJ, Mazhar D. Management of febrile neutropenia in an acute oncology service. *QJM.* 2012;105:327-336.

31 Oberoi S, Trehan A, Marwaha RK, Bansal D. Symptom to door interval in febrile neutropenia: perspective in India. *Support Care Cancer.* 2013;21:1321-1327.

32 Gavidia R, Fuentes SL, Vasquez R, et al. Low socioeconomic status is associated with prolonged times to assessment and treatment, sepsis and infectious death in pediatric fever in El Salvador. *PLoS One.* 2012;7:e43639.

33 Best JT, Frith K, Anderson F, Rapp CG, Rioux L, Ciccarello C. Implementation of an evidence-based order set to impact initial antibiotic time intervals in adult febrile neutropenia. *Oncol Nursing Forum.* 2011;38:661-668.

34 Courtney DM, Aldeen AZ, Gorman SM, et al. Cancer-associated neutropenic fever: clinical outcome and economic costs of emergency department care. *Oncologist.* 2007;12:1019-1026.

35 Pérez Velasco R. Review of granulocyte colony-stimulating factors in the treatment of established febrile neutropenia. *J Oncol Pharm Practice.* 2011;17:225-232.

36 Stanworth SJ, Massey E, Hyde C, et al. Granulocyte transfusions for treating infections in patients with neutropenia or neutrophil dysfunction. *Cochrane Database Syst Rev.* 2005;(3):CD005339.

37 Cherif H, Axdorph U, Kalin M, Björkholm M. Clinical experience of granulocyte transfusion in the management of neutropenic patients with haematological malignancies and severe infection. *Scand J Infect Dis.* 2013;45:112-116.

38 Schimpff SC, Gaya H, Klastersky J, Tattersall MH, Zinner SH. Three antibiotic regimens in the treatment of infection in febrile granulocytopenic patients with cancer. The EORTC international antimicrobial therapy project group. *J Infect Dis.* 1978;137:14-29.

39 Viscoli C, Bruzzi P, Castagnola E, et al. Factors associated with bacteraemia in febrile, granulocytopenic cancer patients. The International Antimicrobial Therapy Cooperative Group (IATCG) of the European Organization for Research and Treatment of Cancer (EORTC). *Eur J Cancer.* 1994;30A:430-437.

40 Flowers CR, Seidenfeld J, Bow EJ, et al. Antimicrobial prophylaxis and outpatient management of fever and neutropenia in adults treated for malignancy: American Society of Clinical Oncology practice guideline. *J Clin Oncol.* 2013;6:794-810.

Chapter 6

Management of persistent fever in patients with neutropenia despite empirical antibiotic administration

The causes of persistent fever

Most patients (85%) receiving empirical antibiotic therapy for febrile neutropenia (FN) will promptly respond with defervescence, especially if predicted at a low risk of complications. The absence of response can be due to resistance of the bacteria or overwhelming bacterial sepsis (especially in non-low-risk patients); these situations pose little diagnostic challenge. The possibility of a noninfectious cause for persistent fever (eg, embolism, drug fever) might be more problematic, although it is a relatively rare event.

Occult fungal infection is a relatively common cause for persistent fever in patients with neutropenia receiving empirical antimicrobial therapy [1]. As summarized in Table 6.1, the incidence of fungal infection in such patients is probably close to 20% [1–6].

The diagnosis of invasive-fungal infections in patients with cancer is notoriously difficult. Attempts have been made to classify these infections on the basis on clinical grounds [7], which is an approach that can be improved by the use of additional biological and radiological diagnostic techniques [6,8]. Nonetheless, because of the difficulty to diagnose invasive-fungal infections in patients with neutropenia, and given the high mortality rate which is associated with such infections,

J. A. Klastersky, *Febrile Neutropenia*,
DOI: 10.1007/978-1-907673-70-2_6, © Springer Healthcare 2014

Incidence of fungal infections in patients with neutropenia not receiving empirical therapy	
Study	**Incidence**
Pizzo et al (1982) [2]	18
EORTC (1989) [3]	28*
Guiot et al (1994) [4]	26*
Corey, Boeckh (2002) [5]	45
Maertens et al (2005) [6]	21

Table 6.1 Incidence of fungal infections in patients with neutropenia not receiving empirical therapy. *Autopsy-based data. Reproduced with permission from © Springer-Verlag 2013, Klastersky et al [1]. All Rights Reserved. Adapted from Pizzo et al [2]; European Organisation for Research and Treatment of Cancer [3]; Guiot et al [4]; Corey, Boeckh [5]; Maertens et al [6].

the therapeutic approach needs to be based on early clinical signs and it should also be broadly designed, as the sensitivity of fungal pathogens is highly variable (and difficult to assess given the frequent and/or late microbiological documentation).

Prevention of invasive-fungal infection

Because of the diagnostic problems and the high mortality rate associated with invasive-fungal infection in persistently neutropenic cancer patients, the prophylactic approach appears sensible and many studies have explored that approach. The traditional use of amphotericin B for such a purpose has been progressively replaced by azoles (fluconazole or voriconazole); although these drugs are more expensive, they have resulted in reduced rates of nephrotoxicity and easier acceptance by the patients, especially in the case of oral administration [9].

More recently, the orally administered posaconazole, a broad-spectrum antifungal agent, was compared to fluconazole or itraconazole as a prophylaxis of invasive-fungal infections in patients undergoing chemotherapy for acute myelogenous leukemia or myelodysplastic syndrome [10]. It was found that posaconazole prevented invasive-fungal infections more effectively than did either fluconazole or itraconazole and improved overall survival. The overall experience with posaconazole for preventing invasive-fungal infections in the context of FN is summarized in Table 6.2; in those patients at a high risk of developing invasive-fungal infections, prophylaxis with posaconazole resulted in an incidence of 0–5% [10–19].

Nonetheless, the use of prophylaxis has drawbacks, such as the emergence of resistant strains; in addition, it makes the drugs used for prophylaxis not suitable for therapeutic purposes. Furthermore, it has been shown that prophylaxis, namely with posaconazole, may reduce the value of negative polymerase chain reaction (PCR) results and delay galactomannan positivity.

Management of suspected invasive-fungal infection

An empirical approach for the management of suspected invasive-fungal infection has been tested in the past due to the relatively high incidence of invasive-fungal infections in persistently febrile and neutropenic patients with cancer as well as the relative difficulty of making a definite diagnosis in many cases, which is associated with high morbidity and

Reference	Years	Type of study	No. pts	No. proven/ probable breakthrough IFDs	Incidence
RCT					
Cornely et al [10]	2002–05	RCT	304	7	2%
"Real life" studies					
Michallet et al [12]	2007–08	Pros	55	2	3.6%
Candoni et al [13]	2009–10	Retro	55	2	4%
Lerolle et al [14]	2007–10	Retro	209	8	3.8%
Egerer et al [15]	2007–09	Retro	76*	1	1.3%
Vehreschild et al [16]	2006–08	Retro	77	3	3.9%
Hahn et al [17]	2007–08	Retro	21	1	5%
Busca et al [18]	2009–10	Retro	61	0	0
Ananda-Rajah et al [19]	2006–10	Retro	68	0	0

Table 6.2 Incidence of proven/probable invasive-fungal diseases in acute myeloid leukemia after posaconazole prophylaxis: data from different types of study. *Number of chemotherapy courses. IFD, invasive-fungal diseases; Pros, prospective study; RCT, randomized clinical trial; Retro, retrospective study. Reproduced with permission from © Ferrata Storti Foundation 2013, Pagano et al [11]. All Rights Reserved. Obtained from Haematologica/the Hematology Journal website http://www.haematologica.org. Adapted from Cornely et al [10]; Michallet et al [12]; Candoni et al [13]; Lerolle et al [14]; Egerer et al [15]; Vehreschild et al [16]; Hahn et al [17]; Busca et al [18]; Ananda-Rajah et al [19].

mortality. A series of collaborative studies conducted by Walsh and colleagues provide extensive and solid information about empirical antifungal therapy [20]. These studies are summarized in Table 6.3 [20]. If we analyze the rates of microbiologically documented failures (ie, breakthrough infections and persistent baseline infections), the failure rates are 13.3% for conventional amphotericin B, 8.2% for liposomal amphotericin B, 3.5% for voriconazole, and 7.7% for caspofungin. Moreover, it was shown that conventional amphotericin B was less tolerated than the other regimens in terms of nephrotoxicity and infusion-related events; both voriconazole and caspofungin were better tolerated than liposomal amphotericin B. Based on these data, the incidence of invasive-fungal infection in patients with persistent FN is 20%, and it can thus be concluded that the empirical use of voriconazole or caspofungin reduces invasive-fungal infection in these patients to less than 5%, with minimal toxicity.

However, the concept of using empirical therapy for possible invasive-fungal infection implies giving broad spectrum antifungal agents to all patients with persistent FN, which may result in overtreatment, with potentially toxic and expensive drugs. Thus, it is not surprising that the so-called "preemptive" approach has been proposed [24]. The preemptive approach suggests that by using biological and radiological evidence in selected groups of patients with FN, clinicians may be able to limit the overtreatment associated with empirical antifungal therapy, without jeopardizing the clinical effectiveness.

A randomized controlled trial compared empirical versus preemptive antifungal therapy for high-risk patients with FN [25]. Probable and proven invasive-fungal infection were more common among patients who received preemptive treatment than among patients who received empirical therapy (13 out of 143 vs 4 out of 150; $p<0.05$). Preemptive therapy did not reduce the risk of nephrotoxicity but decreased the cost of antifungal therapy by 35%. Thus, the option between empiric versus preemptive therapy of probable invasive-fungal infections in predisposed patients with FN is not yet entirely settled [26]. Empirical therapy bears the risk of overtreatment but preemptive therapy may sometimes be initiated too late to be fully effective.

Measures of the success of empirical antifungal therapy with conventional or liposomal amphotericin B, voriconazole, or caspofungin

Variable	Conventional amphotericin B*	Liposomal amphotericin B*			Voriconazole†	Caspofungin‡
		Versus conventional amphotericin B*	Versus voriconazole†	Versus caspofungin‡		
No. of patients	344	343	422	539	415	556
Overall success (% of patients)	49.4	50.1	30.6	33.7	26.0	33.9
Resolution of fever (% of patients)	58.1	58.0	36.5	41.4	32.5	41.2
No. breakthrough fungal infection (% of patients)	89.2	90.1	95.0	95.5	98.1	94.8
Resolution of baseline fungal infection (% of patients)	72.7	81.8	66.7	25.9	46.2	51.9
Survival for 7 days (% of patients)	89.5	92.7	94.1	89.2	92.0	92.6
No discontinuation because of toxic effects (% of patients)	81.4	85.7	93.4	85.5	90.1	89.7

* The data are from Walsh et al, 1999 [21]
† The data are from Walsh et al, 2002 [22]
‡ The data are from Walsh et al, 2004 [23]

Table 6.3 Measures of the success of empirical antifungal therapy with conventional or liposomal amphotericin B, voriconazole, or caspofungin. Reproduced with permission from © Massachusetts Medical Society 2013, Klastersky et al [20]. All Rights Reserved. Adapted from Walsh et al [21]; Walsh et al [22]; Walsh et al [23].

It is of great importance to better predict which patients are at risk for developing invasive-fungal infections and to provide specific prophylaxis to them. In case of persistent fever, in spite of antibiotic administration, empirical antifungal treatment should be administered in most high-risk patients.

Therapy of established invasive-fungal infections

A recent, large, observational, prospective study in which 59% of the patients were treated early, liposomal amphotericin B and caspofungin were the most common single-agent therapies. The 12-week mortality rate was 18% for probable/proven aspergillosis, 15% for proven candidiasis, 10% for probable/proven invasive-fungal infections, 9% for possible invasive infections, and 3% for FN [27]. Based on these data, the mortality for proven candidiasis and aspergillosis remains relatively high, and it thus seems appropriate to increase efforts to document these infections as often as possible via blood cultures, broncho–alveolar lavages, and biopsies in order to orient therapy to be as specific as possible.

Current recommendations for treatment of candidemia and invasive candidiasis in patients with neutropenia include echinocandins and liposomal amphotericin B as well as triazoles in less critically ill patients. Recent data from a systematic review of randomized controlled trials suggest a trend toward better outcomes with the use of non-amphotericin agents, although the results did not reach statistical significance [28]. Across these studies, echinocandins were most beneficial in terms of favorable outcomes with the fewest side effects and toxicity. However, it is important to note the epidemiology of candidiasis in each given institution when selecting the options for empirical therapy prior to microbiological identification. This is especially true in terms of susceptibility to antifungal agents, which can be greatly influenced by the local prescription habits and the often-used prophylaxis in predisposed patients.

Aspergillus species have emerged as an important cause of life-threatening infections, especially in patients with prolonged neutropenia. The Infectious Diseases Society of America recently provided comprehensive guidelines for managing aspergillar infections [29]. In a large, randomized, controlled trial, voriconazole was shown to be superior to deoxycholate amphotericin B and is thus recommended for the primary treatment of suspected invasive aspergillosis; liposomal amphotericin B is being considered as an alternative primary therapy for some patients. Salvage therapy for invasive aspergillosis poses important challenges, especially in patients in which aspergillosis is resistant to voriconazole; not much evidence-based data exist to guide management.

Besides candidiasis and aspergillosis, a series of other invasive-fungal infections, with distinctive clinical and microbiological characteristics, do constantly emerge. A special challenge is represented by the variability of their susceptibility to antifungal agents, making the choice of empirical therapy more difficult. There is a definite place for careful antimicrobial stewardship here in order to accelerate diagnosis, evaluate susceptibility to available agents, and provide the optimal therapeutic guidelines.

References

1   Klastersky J, Paesmans M. Antifungal therapy in febrile neutropenic patients: review of treatment choices and strategies for aspergillar infection. *Support Care Cancer.* 2007;15:137-141.

2   Pizzo PA, Robichaud KJ, Gill FA, Witebsky FG. Empiric antibiotic and antifungal therapy for cancer patients with prolonged fever and granulocytopenia. *Am J Med.* 1982;72:101-111.

3   European Organisation for Research and Treatment of Cancer, International Antimicrobial Therapy Cooperative Group. Empiric antifungal therapy in febrile granulocytopenic patients. *Am J Med.* 1989;86:668-672.

4   Guiot HFL, Fibbe WE, Van't Wout JW. Risk factors for fungal infection in patients with malignant hematologic disorders: implications for empirical therapy and prophylaxis. *Clin Infect Dis.* 1994;18:525-532.

5   Corey L, Boeckh M. Persistent fever in patients with neutropenia. *N Engl J Med.* 2002;346:222-224.

6   Maertens J, Theunissen K, Verhoef G, et al. Galactomannan and computed tomography-based preemptive antifungal therapy in neutropenic patients at high risk for invasive fungal infection: a prospective feasibility study. *Clin Infect Dis.* 2005;41:1242-1250.

7   Ascioglu S, Rex JH, de Pauw B, et al; Invasive Fungal Infections Cooperative Group of the European Organization for Research and Treatment of Cancer; Mycoses Study Group of the National Institute of Allergy and Infectious Diseases. Defining opportunistic invasive fungal infections in immunocompromised patients with cancer and hematopoietic stem cell transplants: an international consensus. *Clin Infect Dis.* 2002;34:7-14.

8   Cuenca-Estrella M, Meije Y, Diaz-Pedroche C, et al. Value of serial quantification of fungal DNA by a real-time PCR-based technique for early diagnosis of invasive aspergillosis in patients with febrile neutropenia. *J Clin Microbiol.* 2009;47:379-384.

9   Riedel A, Choe L, Inciardi J, Yuen C, Martin T, Guglielmo BJ. Antifungal prophylaxis in chemotherapy-associated neutropenia: a restrospective, observational study. *BMC Infect Dis.* 2007;7:70.

10 Cornely OA, Maertens J, Winston DJ, et al. Posaconazole vs. fluconazole or itraconazole prophylaxis in patients with neutropenia. *N Engl J Med.* 2007;356:348-359.

11 Pagano L, Caira M, Cuenca-Estrella M. The management of febrile neutropenia in the posaconazole era: a new challenge? *Haematologica*. 2012;97:963-965.

12 Michallet M, Sobh M, Morisset S, et al. Risk factors for invasive aspergillosis in acute myeloid leukemia patients prophylactically treated with posaconazole. *Med Mycol*. 2011;49:681-687.

13 Candoni A, Simeone E, Caira M, Mazzuzzo M, Fanin R, Pagano L. Prophylaxis of invasive fungal diseases with posaconazole in acute myeloid leukemia. A real life experience. Abstract O804 at 16th EHA (European Hematology Association) Congress; June 11, 2011.

14 Lerolle N, Lafaurie M, Touratier S, et al. Breakthrough invasive fungal infections in patients with hematological cancers receiving posaconazole prophylaxis: a four-year study. Abstract M-1521 ICAAC; Chicago. Sept. 2011.

15 Egerer G, Geist MJ. Posaconazole prophylaxis in patients with acute myelogenous leukaemia--results from an observational study. *Mycoses*. 2011;54(Suppl 1):7-11.

16 Vehreschild JJ, Rüping MJ, Wisplinghoff H, et al. Clinical effectiveness of posaconazole prophylaxis in patients with acute myelogenous leukaemia: a 6 year experience of the Cologne AML cohort. *J Antimicrob Chemother*. 2010;65:1466-1471.

17 Hahn J, Stifel F, Reichle A, Holler E, Andreesen R. Clinical experience with posaconazole prophylaxis--a retrospective analysis in a haematological unit. *Mycoses*. 2011;54(Suppl 1):12-16.

18 Busca A, Frairia C, Marmont F, et al. Posaconazole vs standard azoles for prevention of invasive fungal infections in patients with acute myeloid leukemia. Poster P088 at 5th TIMM (Trends in Medical Mycology) Congress; Valencia. Oct 2–5, 2011.

19 Ananda-Rajah MR, Grigg A, Downey MT, et al. Comparative clinical effectiveness of prophylactic voriconazole/posaconazole to fluconazole/itraconazole in patients with acute myeloid leukaemia/myelodysplastic syndrome undergoing cytotoxic chemotherapy over a 12-year period. *Haematologica*. 2012;97:459-463.

20 Klastersky J. Antifungal therapy in patients with fever and neutropenia – More rational and less empirical? *N Engl J Med*. 2004;351:1445-1447.

21 Walsh TJ, Finberg RW, Arndt C, et al. Liposomal amphotericin B for empirical therapy in patients with persistent fever and neutropenia. National Institute of Allergy and Infectious Diseases Mycoses Study Group. *N Engl J Med*. 1999;340:764-771.

22 Walsh TJ, Pappas P, Winston DJ, et al; National Institute of Allergy and Infectious Diseases Mycoses Study Group. Voriconazole compared with liposomal amphotericin B for empirical antifungal therapy in patients with neutropenia and persistent fever. *N Engl J Med*. 2002;346:225-234.

23 Walsh TJ, Teppler H, Donowitz GR, et al. Caspofungin versus liposomal amphotericin B for empirical antifungal therapy in patients with persistent fever and neutropenia. *N Engl J Med*. 2004;351:1391-1402.

24 Maertens J, Deeren D, Dierickx D, Theunissen K. Preemptive antifungal therapy: still a way to go. *Curr Opin Infect Dis*. 2006;19:551-556.

25 Cordonnier C, Pautas C, Maury S, et al. Empirical versus antifungal therapy for high-risk, febrile, neutropenic patients: a randomized, controlled trial. *Clin Infect Dis*. 2009;48:1042-1051.

26 Rieger CT, Ostermann H. Empiric vs preemptive antifungal treatment: an appraisal of treatment strategies in haematological patients. *Mycoses*. 2008;51:(Suppl 1):31-34.

27 Herbrecht R, Caillot D, Cordonnier C, et al. Indications and outcomes of antifungal therapy in French patients with haematological conditions or recipients of haematopoietic stem cell transplantation. *J Antimicrob Chemother*. 2012;67:2731-2738.

28 Kanji JN, Laverdière M, Rotstein C, Walsh TJ, Shah PS, Haider S. Treatment of invasive candidiasis in neutropenic patients: systematic review of randomized controlled treatment trials. *Leuk Lymphoma*. 2013;54:1479-1487.

29 Walsh TJ, Anaissie EJ, Denning DW, et al; Infectious Diseases Society of America. Treatment of aspergillosis: clinical practice guidelines of the Infectious Diseases Society of America. *Clin Infect Dis*. 2008;46:327-360.

Chapter 7

Costs associated with febrile neutropenia

General conditions

Evaluation of costs associated with a medical condition and cost effectiveness of therapy do not usually take into account the indirect harm that the condition causes in terms of deterioration of the quality of life. Febrile neutropenia (FN) is an illness requiring antimicrobial therapy and possible hospitalization, often disturbing the familial and social life; it may lead to reduction, delay, or even discontinuation of effective chemotherapy, causing thus a direct prejudice to the patient's health.

It should be stressed that the cost of medical care is very different from country to country, which makes generalizations difficult in this following chapter.

Magnitude of the costs associated with febrile neutropenia

A recent study from the USA [1] shows that patients with FN incurred greater costs (9628 USD per patient/month) than cancer patients without FN (8478 USD per patient/month). In patients with FN, hospitalization accounted for 53% of the costs while chemotherapy comprised the majority of costs in patients without FN. Patients with FN who died had the highest mean total costs compared to patients with FN who survived (24,214 USD vs 8227 USD per patient/month). Additionally, the majority of FN episodes (79%) occurred during the first chemotherapy course and the average costs for FN were highest for inpatients (22,086 USD)

J. A. Klastersky, *Febrile Neutropenia*,
DOI: 10.1007/978-1-907673-70-2_7, © Springer Healthcare 2014

compared to outpatients (985 USD); this difference was observed for most of the common tumor types (colorectal, non-Hodgkin's lymphoma, ovarian, breast, and lung cancer).

Another retrospective study from the USA analyzed the costs and outcome associated with hospitalized cancer patients with FN [2]. The mean hospitalization costs were 18,042 USD for patients with neutropenia, 22,839 USD for those with FN, and 27,587 USD for patients with neutropenia and documented infection; mortality rates followed a similar trend: 8.3%, 13.7%, and 19.4%, respectively. It was concluded that cancer patients with FN are causing high inpatient hospitalization costs that actually exceed those previously reported.

In the late 1990s, a cost-minimization model utilizing cost and effectiveness concluded that the use of myeloid growth factors lowered the expenses when the risk of hospitalization was over 22% (Figure 7.1) [3,4]. This cut-off was based on an estimated daily cost of hospitalization for FN of between 1675 USD and 1892 USD. At the above threshold, the cost of treating FN occurrence was greater than the expense of primary myeloid growth factors prophylaxis. This led to the wide acceptance of a 20% threshold for the risk of developing FN in order to decide whether or not the administration of primary prophylaxis with myeloid growth factors was indicated.

These recommendations should be, nonetheless, critically analyzed. First, the costs of FN are probably underestimated and should be adapted to the present day situation; it might make the cost effectiveness of the myeloid growth factors primary prophylaxis look better. However, since hospitalization is no longer the rule for many patients with FN, this may make primary prophylaxis look less cost effective.

Reducing the cost of febrile neutropenia
Home therapy for febrile neutropenia
A recent study from Australia [5] analyses the cost of FN in ambulatory versus in-hospital settings. Two strategies for ambulatory care were studied in patients with a low risk of complications during FN (using a modified Multinational Association for Supportive Care in Cancer [MASCC] score): (1) outpatient care for the entire episode of FN or

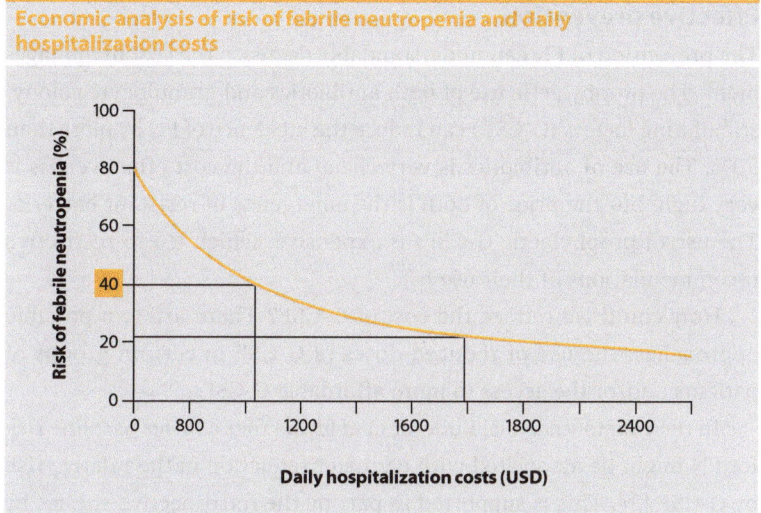

Figure 7.1 Economic analysis of risk of febrile neutropenia and daily hospitalization costs. Adapted from Lyman et al [3]. Reproduced with permission from © Springer 2013, Hirsch, Lyman [4]. All Rights Reserved.

(2) early discharge after a brief hospitalization (at least 24 hours) for patient evaluation and initial monitoring of symptoms, followed by outpatient care. Compared to the current standard of care in Australia (ie, inpatient hospitalization), the weighted average cost savings per episode of low-risk FN was 35% for outpatient follow-up only and 30% for early discharge and outpatient follow-up.

Ambulatory care for low-risk patients with FN is probably cost effective if compared to inpatient care for the same patients. Nonetheless, it should be stressed that the bulk of the costs for FN is devoted to those patients who are not at low risk and who present serious complications requiring extensive and sometimes aggressive medical support; plus, patients with FN who die account for the greatest healthcare costs [1]. Thus, the outpatient approach for the low-risk patients will probably not have a major impact on the improvement of cost effectiveness. Moreover, it may be speculated that the size of the non-low-risk population of patients with FN will progressively increase in the future, as the overall population is getting older; age being a recognized factor which increases the risk of complications during an episode of FN [6].

Effective prevention

The prevention of FN can understandably decrease the cost of management. The prophylactic use of both antibiotics and granulocyte colony-stimulating factors (G-CSF) can reduce the incidence of FN by more than 50%. The use of antibiotics is very cheap and the cost effectiveness is very high, but the price of both is the emergence of resistant bacteria. The use of prophylactic G-CSFs is expensive, which led to restrictive recommendations of their use [6].

How could we reduce the cost of G-CSF? There are two possible approaches: the use of reduced doses of G-CSF in certain groups of patients and/or the access to more affordable G-CSFs.

In their meta-analysis, Kuderer et al found that a lower baseline risk for FN might be associated with a greater reduction in the relative risk by G-CSF [7]. This is supported in part by the retrospective studies by Papaldo et al [8] where the administration of a reduced dose of G-CSF was as active as more intensive regimens in patients with a relatively low risk of developing FN. Whether the indications for the use of G-CSF should be extended to those patients with a low risk of FN is debatable [9] but might be considered as these patients (eg, elderly and having various comorbidities) represent a large proportion of the patients receiving chemotherapy today. Moreover, once FN occurs in those patients, the resulting morbidity and mortality is similar to those seen in patients at a higher risk for developing FN [10].

The other approach to optimize the cost effectiveness of G-CSFs would be to significantly decrease their cost. This is achievable now through the introduction of biosimilar G-CSFs, which seems to be comparable in efficacy to the original products [11]. There is evidence that biosimilar G-CSFs are as active as the original compounds and are sold at about 60% of their price, showing a clear cost advantage.

In fact, these two approaches for extending the indications of prophylactic G-CSF might be theoretically combined: that is, both reducing the dosage and using a more affordable biosimilar to achieve cost effectiveness in a population of patients with cancer at a relatively low risk of developing FN [12].

Thus, a new type of algorithm might be proposed for the prevention of FN and its consequences in a larger proportion of patients with cancer at risk of FN, without compromising the cost effectiveness of such an approach (Figure 7.2) [12]. These propositions should of course be verified in adequately designed and conducted clinical trials.

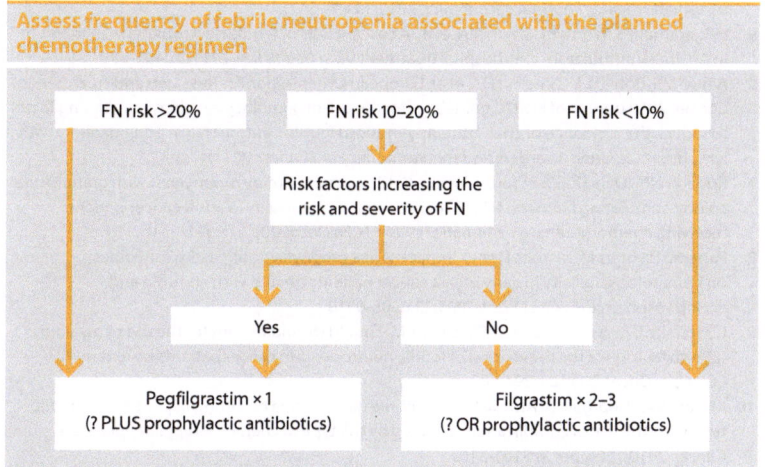

Figure 7.2 Assess frequency of febrile neutropenia associated with the planned chemotherapy regimen. FN, febrile neutropenia. Reproduced with permission from © Karger AG 2013, Klastersky, Paesmans [12]. All Rights Reserved.

References

1 Michels SL, Barron RL, Reynolds MW, Smoyer Tomic K, Yu J, Lyman GH. Costs associated with febrile neutropenia in the US. *Pharmacoeconomics*. 2012;30:809-823.
2 Schilling MB, Parks C, Deeter RG. Costs and outcomes associated with hospitalized cancer patients with neutropenic complications: a retrospective study. *Exp Ther Med*. 2011;2:859-866.
3 Lyman GH, Kuderer N, Greene J, Balducci L. The economics of febrile neutropenia: implications for the use of colony-stimulating factors. *Eur J Cancer*. 1998;34:1857-1864.
4 Hirsch BR, Lyman GH. Pharmacoeconomics of the myeloid growth factors. A critical and systematic review. *Pharmacoeconomics*. 2012;30:497-511.
5 Lingaratnam S, Worth LJ, Slavin MA, et al. A cost analysis of febrile neutropenia management in Australia: ambulatory v. in-hospital treatment. *Aust Health Rev*. 2011;35:491-500.
6 Aapro MS, Bohlius J, Cameron DA, et al; European Organisation for Research and Treatment of Cancer. 2010 update of EORTC guidelines for the use of granulocyte-colony stimulating factor to reduce the incidence of chemotherapy-induced febrile neutropenia in adult patients with lymphoproliferative disorders and solid tumours. *Eur J Cancer*. 2011;47:8-32.
7 Kuderer NM, Dale DC, Crawford J, Lyman GH. Impact of primary prophylaxis with granulocyte colony-stimulating factor on febrile neutropenia and mortality in adult cancer patients receiving chemotherapy: a systematic review. *J Clin Oncol*. 2007;25:3158-3167.
8 Papaldo P, Lopez M, Marolla P, et al. Impact of five prophylactic filgrastim schedules on hematologic toxicity in early breast cancer patients treated with epirubin and cyclophosphamide. *J Clin Oncol*. 2005;23:6908-6918.
9 Klastersky J, Awada A, Aoun M, Paesmans M. Should the indications for the use of myeloid growth factors for the prevention of febrile neutropenia in cancer patients be extended? *Curr Opin Oncol*. 2009;21:297-302.
10 Klastersky J, Georgala A, Ameye L, et al. Febrile neutropenia occurring in patients with solid tumors: is the risk of complications affected by the type of chemotherapy? *Support Care Cancer*. 2010;18(Suppl 3):S101-S102.
11 Hadji P, Kostev K, Schröder-Bernhardi D, Ziller V. Cost comparison of outpatient treatment with granulocyte colony-stimulating factors (G-CSF) in Germany. *Int J Clin Pharmacol Ther*. 2012;50:281-289.
12 Klastersky JA, Paesmans M. Treatment of febrile neutropenia is expensive: prevention is the answer. *Onkologie*. 2011;34:226-228.

Chapter 8

At the extremes of age: febrile neutropenia in children and elderly

Febrile neutropenia in the pediatric population

The criteria for diagnosing febrile neutropenia (FN) in children are not different from those used in adults. Slight modifications of the definition – such as the inclusion of a high fever – were not associated with a change of the rate of FN or FN-associated with bacteremia [1].

There is no established consensus for the predictive significance of biological parameters in terms of diagnosis or prognosis of severe complications of FN in children, which is also true for adults. However, a series of studies have evaluated different markers of inflammation as predictive of different types of infection, with variable conclusions. These included procalcitonin, interleukin (IL)-6, IL-8, C-reactive protein (CRP), and others. Currently, it seems that IL-6 may help differentiate patients with fever of unknown origin (FUO) from children with documented infections, and that a rising CRP might be indicative of serious infection [2]. In contrast with adult patients, it is possible that repeating blood cultures in children with persistent FN, even when several initial blood cultures have been negative, may identify patients with serious bacterial infections and allow for earlier targeted therapy of these infections [3].

Evidence-based guidelines for the management of pediatric FN have been recently proposed [4]. Some recommendations are similar to those of adult guidelines (eg, choice of empirical regimens and their subsequent modifications). Some other recommendations, such as oral antibacterial

J. A. Klastersky, *Febrile Neutropenia*,
DOI: 10.1007/978-1-907673-70-2_8, © Springer Healthcare 2014

therapy and outpatient management, have been adapted to the specific needs of the pediatric population.

In contrast, there are more conspicuous differences in the proposed risk-stratification schema, which are presented as "pediatric specific", and in some of the diagnostic tools, such as beta-D-glucan galactomannan assays. With respect to the definition of a "low-risk" pediatric group, a recent study (Delphi survey) proposed a national (UK) framework for identification and managements of children with FN [5].

There is a definite need to build specific algorithms suitable for the pediatric population, namely in the areas of risk stratification and cost effectiveness [6] because:

1. Pediatric cancers differ from adult neoplasia in terms of both nature and therapeutic approach.
2. There are physiological differences between children and adults.
3. Lastly, specific psychological and social methods must be used for children, which differ from those used for adults.

Febrile neutropenia in the elderly

For the selection of anticancer therapy, several studies indicate that there is a clear age effect beyond the impact of comorbidity. Also, the selected elderly patients who are enrolled in anticancer strategies tend to have a similar benefit from their treatment at the cost of a similar or somewhat higher toxicity [7].Geriatric assessment can provide more crucial information regarding the affect of a patient's age beyond what could be learned from classical oncological prognostic factors, such as the Eastern Cooperative Oncology Group (ECOG) performance status scale. A geriatric assessment can identify many problems in older patients with cancer, add pragmatic information, and may improve outcomes.

Hematopoiesis in elderly patients is somewhat less efficient than in younger patients; blood stem-cell populations may decrease and regulation of hematopoiesis is jeopardized by modified cytokine expression [8]. Therefore, in terms of myelosuppression, several studies found higher age to be a general risk factor for the development of severe neutropenia and neutropenia-related complications. Because most older patients can derive the same benefit from aggressive chemotherapy as younger patients, it is important to address the risks of neutropenia in a specific way in older patients to make the administration of full-dose chemotherapy possible [9]. From these considerations – the progressively impaired hematopoiesis with age and the potential benefit of full-dose chemotherapy in elderly patients – it is imperative that a special emphasis should be put on the prevention of FN in elderly patients.

The Elderly Task Force of the European Organisation for Research and Treatment of Cancer (EORTC) conducted a detailed literature search (1992–2002) to derive evidence-based conclusions on the value of pro-phylactic administration of granulocyte colony-stimulating factor (G-CSF) in elderly patients receiving chemotherapy [10]. They found that the use of prophylactic G-CSF allowed for:

- the administration of planned, scheduled doses of chemotherapy,
- reduced the incidence of chemotherapy-induced FN, and
- reduced serious infections in a variety of tumors in elderly patients.

The authors concluded that pegfilgrastim should be used prophylacti-cally in elderly patients (>65 years) to support the optimal delivery of standard therapy. These recommendations have been endorsed by the EORTC guidelines for the use of G-CSF [11]; more specific recommenda-tions for the most common hematological cancers in the elderly have been recently reviewed [9] and are probably applicable to most situations in patients with solid-tumor cancers who also derive the same benefit from chemotherapy, as do younger patients. However, as stressed in a recent study comparing the relative effectiveness and safety of chemotherapy in elderly and non-elderly patients with advanced colon cancer, the grade III and IV adverse events resulting from chemotherapy are more frequent in elderly patients [12]. Therefore, these complications should be anticipated and aggressively prevented and treated.

The Multinational Association of Supportive Care in Cancer (MASCC) score index takes age into account when assessing the risk stratification of FN [13]. However, oral therapy plus early discharge policy should be implemented more cautiously in older patients presenting with FN, although this needs to be validated in adequate clinical trials.

It was actually found that older patients with FN were more likely than the younger patients to receive inappropriate antibiotic therapy and other supportive measures [14]. The choice of antibacterial therapy should take into account several key points that commonly affect the elderly:

- the frequently impaired renal function in elderly patients;
- emesis and mucositis are often more severe in elderly patients, and thus adequate hydration should be provided throughout the febrile episode; and
- the thirst mechanisms may be decreased in the elderly.

Admission to the intensive care unit is often proposed with reluctance to older patients with neoplasia. However, if the decision has been made to give chemotherapy to such patients, it is clearly the ethical responsibility of the treating physician to provide full support in case of any chemotherapy-induced toxicity, namely FN.

A recent study has shown that almost half of the patients with hematological malignancies and life-threatening complications can be discharged safely from the intensive care unit and that age or underlying characteristics do not influence the outcome [15]. Thus, in an elderly patient with chemotherapy-induced FN, the admission to the intensive care unit for surveillance and possibly early therapy should be considered more often and even earlier than in younger patients, rather than the opposite.

We have limited evidence-based information on how to manage FN in elderly patients. This is mainly due to the fact that it was not until recently that elderly patients with cancer were treated with the same methods as younger patients. Thus, until now, elderly patients were often excluded from clinical trials. Nonetheless, some recommendations can be made (Table 8.1) and be tested in adequately designed trials.

Pragmatic recommendation for the management of febrile neutropenia in elderly patients (>65 years)
Provide primary G-CSF prophylaxis to all patients unless the risk of FN is minimal (<5%)
For patients with FN, provide assessment and empiric therapy on an emergency basis
For low-risk patients, use the oral antibiotics/early discharge with great caution; favor surveillance
For non-low-risk patients, consider early admission to intensive care unit for surveillance and early appropriate measures as needed

Table 8.1 Pragmatic recommendation for the management of febrile neutropenia in elderly patients (>65 years). FN, febrile neutropenia; G-CSF, granulocyte colony-stimulating factor.

References

1. Binz P, Bodmer N, Leibundgut K, Teuffel O, Niggli FK, Ammann RA. Different fever definitions and the rate of fever and neutropenia diagnosed in children with cancer: a retrospective two-center cohort study. *Pediatr Blood Cancer.* 2012;60:799-805.

2. Chaudhary N, Kosaraju K, Bhat K, Bairy I, Borker A. Significance of interleukin-6 (IL-6) and C-reactive protein (CRP) in children and young adults with febrile neutropenia during chemotherapy for cancer: a prospective study. *J Pediatr Hematol Oncol.* 2012;34:617-623.

3. Rosenblum J, Lin J, Kim M, Levy AS. Repeating blood cultures in neutorpenic children with persistent fevers when the initial blood culture is negative. *Pediatr Blood Cancer.* 2013;60:923-927.

4. Lehrnbecker T, Phillips R, Alexander S, et al; International Pediatric Fever and Neutropenia Guideline Panel. Guideline for the management of fever and neutropenia in children with cancer and/or undergoing hematopietic stem-cell transplantation. *J Clin Oncol.* 2012;30:4427-4438.

5. Gibson F, Chisholm J, Brandford E, et al; CCLG Supportive Care Group. Developing a national 'low risk' febrile neutropenia framework for use in children and young people's cancer care. *Support Care Cancer.* 2013;5:1241-1251.

6. Pulsipher MA. Pediatric-specific guidelines for fever and neutropenia: a catalyst for improving care and focusing research. *J Clin Oncol.* 2012;35:4292-4293.

7. Exsesmann M. Geriatric oncology: an overview of progresses and challenges. *Cancer Res Treat.* 2010;42:61-68.

8. Gillison TL, Chatta GS. Cancer chemotherapy in the elderly patient. *Oncology (Williston Park).* 2010;24:76-85.

9. Klastersky J, Gombos A, Georgala A, Awada A. Prevention of neutropenia-related events in elderly patients with hematological cancer. *Aging Health.* 2011;7:829-842.

10. Repetto L, Biganzoli L, Koehne CH, et al. EORTC Cancer in the Elderly Task Force guidelines for the use of colony-stimulating factors in elderly patients with cancer. *Eur J Cancer.* 2003;39:2264-2272.

11. Aapro MS, Cameron DA, Pessengell R, et al; European Organisation for Research and Treatment of Cancer (EORTC) Granulocyte Colony-Stimulating Factor (G-CSF) Guidelines Working Party. EORTC guidelines for the use of granulocyte-colony stimulating factor to reduce the incidence of chemotherapy-induced febrile neutropenia in adult patients with lymphomas and solid tumours. *Eur J Cancer.* 2006;42:2433-2453.

12. Lyman GH, Lyman CH, Agboola O. Risk models for predicting chemotherapy-induced neutropenia. *Oncologist.* 2005;10:427-437.

13. Hung A, Mullins CD. Relative effectiveness and safety of chemotherapy in elderly and nonelderly patients with stage III colon cancer: a systematic review. *Oncologist.* 2013;1:54-63.

14. Klastersky J, Paesmans M, Rubenstein EB, et al. The multinational Association for Supporting Care in Cancer risk index: a multinational scoring system for identifying low-risk febrile neutropenic cancer patients. *J Clin Oncol.* 2000;18:3038-3051.

15. Nørgaard M, Larsson H, Pedersen G, Schønheyder HC, Rothman KJ, Sørensen HT. Short-term mortality of bacteraemia in elderly patients with haematological malignancies. *Br J Haematol.* 2005;32:25-31.